MW00510987

Keto Diet Recipes

Low Carb and Ketogenic Diet Recipes for Healthy Living.
Enjoy the Keto Lifestyle with Quick, Easy and Delicious Recipes to Lose Weight, Lower cholesterol and Reverse Diabetes. Keto Life Guide.

Alexangel Kitchen

Just for Our Readers

To Thank You for Purchasing the Book, for a limited time, you can get a Special FREE BOOK from Alexangel Kitchen

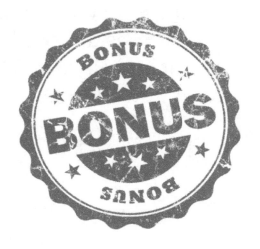

Just go to https://alexangelkitchen.com/ to download your FREE BOOK

COPYRIGHT

© Copyright 2021 all right reserved by Yurino

This document is geared towards providing exact and reliable information with regard to the topic and issue covered. The publication is sold with the idea that the publisher is not required to render accounting, officially permitted or otherwise qualified services. If advice is necessary, legal or professional, a practiced individual in the profession should be ordered.

- From a Declaration of Principles which was accepted and approved equally by a Committee of the American Bar Association and a Committee of Publishers and Associations.

In no way is it legal to reproduce, duplicate, or transmit any part of this document in either electronic means or in printed format. Recording of this publication is strictly prohibited, and any storage of this document is not allowed unless with written permission from the publisher. All rights reserved.

The information provided herein is stated to be truthful and consistent, in that any liability, in terms of inattention or otherwise, by any usage or abuse of any policies, processes, or directions contained within is the solitary and utter responsibility of the recipient reader. Under no circumstances will any legal responsibility or blame be held against the publisher for any reparation, damages, or monetary loss due to the information herein, either directly or indirectly.

Respective authors own all copyrights not held by the publisher.

The information herein is offered for informational purposes solely and is universal as so. The presentation of the information is without contract or any type of guarantee assurance.

The trademarks that are used are without any consent, and the publication of the trademark is without permission or backing by the trademark owner. All trademarks and brands within this book are for clarifying purposes only and are owned by the owners themselves, not affiliated with this document.

Table of Contents

INTRODUCTION

When thinking about a diet or change in lifestyle, it's critical to think about the advantages and entanglements. If the diet won't profit you – what's the point? Yet additionally, if the symptoms are unmanageable, you might need to reconsider. Keto diets are more well-known than any time in recent memory with a high number of competitors changing to along these lines of eating/living. The Keto diet/method for living comprises of eating nourishments that are high in fat, moderate in protein and low in carbs. When on a Keto diet, the body adjusts from utilizing carbs to utilizing fats to consume vitality.

Here we take a gander at the advantages of the Keto diet, and for what reason is may be for you. Remember to find out about the reactions as well – we couldn't not have a reasonable contention, might we be able to!

1 – Improved body organization

Obviously, one of the principle reasons that individuals move to any diet is to improve their body shape and piece. The Keto diet has been demonstrated to diminish muscle versus fat and build fit weight, basically making somebody look more slender. When combined with quality preparing and lifting, the body organization can improve most prominently.

2 – Increased vitality levels

When you eat heaps of carbs for the duration of the day, your glucose levels go here and there. On the Keto diet, your vitality levels are bound to be reliable for the duration of the day as you're not getting the spikes in glucose. The perpetual stock of vitality from the high fats are probably going to keep you feeling stimulated and will stop those spikes. It is critical to call attention to however that when beginning on a Keto diet, your vitality levels might be lower because of weariness from the stun to your collection of eating less carbs.

3 – Can decrease awful skin

Eating a Keto diet has been demonstrated to help diminish skin inflammation and awful skin. As the Keto diet removes carbs and prepared nourishments which can have effect on gut health, many notice an improvement to their skin on this diet.

4 – Reduces cholesterol

Studies have discovered that the Keto diet can help decrease cholesterol and can make your heart healthier. Great cholesterol levels have been seen as expanded on the Keto diet, with terrible cholesterol being decreased.

5 – Reduces pulse

Low carb diets like the Keto Diet have been demonstrated to decrease pulse. Studies have demonstrated that eating less carbs can significantly affect decreasing this.

6 – Reduced fat particles in the body

Fat particles, otherwise called triglycerides will in general decrease drastically when on the Keto Diet. Expanded fat particles are often determined via starch utilization and fructose (sugar). When individuals cut carbs, their fat atoms significantly decrease. In actuality, when individuals cut fats in their diet, fat particles can really increment. This isn't an issue on the Keto diet which is high in fats.

7 – Reduced possibility of coronary illness

Instinctive fat will be fat under the skin in the stomach pit which lodges itself around the organs and can be hurtful. Low carb diets help to decrease instinctive fat, particularly that around the stomach pit. In the long haul, having less fat around there can lessen the danger of coronary illness and furthermore type 2 diabetes.

There are numerous advantages of going to a Keto Diet, yet recollect that this sort of diet ought to be considered as a long haul lifestyle change and not a prevailing fashion diet. The Keto diet is commended by numerous individuals for its outcomes in fat decrease and can likewise help with numerous other health upgrades.

KETO DIET RECIPES

You should seriously mull over diet a no-no on a ketogenic diet — yet reconsider. These keto diet recipes catch the equivalent springy, chewy, and toasty surface as common portions, all while keeping you all the more full and centered.

The most effective method to make the best keto diet

When getting ready keto diet recipes, pay special mind to low-carb ingredients that could add to brain haze and aggravation. Skip recipes that require regular dairy or yeast, and abstain from eating basic keto diet ingredients like psyllium husk, thickener, and nuts or nut margarines time after time — these can contain shape or disturb your gut. Grass-encouraged margarine, ghee, and coconut flour are the couple of exemptions that will at present produce an excellent portion.
From great cut diet to tortillas and sweet portions, keep these keto diet recipes close by for all your hardest carb desires:

Essential Keto Diet Recipes

This elastic, supplement stuffed portion utilizes heat-safe collagen peptides to give each chomp an additional protein support. With extra ingredients like almond flour and eggs, this formula makes a durable cut that holds up to sandwiches and spreads. In contrast to most recipes, this keto diet is an extraordinary 0 net carbs!

10

This collagen keto diet has zero net carbs per cut. It's sans dairy, sans grain, sans gluten, and the best part is that it utilizes heat-stable, grass-bolstered collagen protein as its essential element for giving the diet its structure. This keto diet is feathery, tasty, not excessively eggy, and this with zero net carbs per cut.

This keto diet formula is so natural to work with that the conceivable outcomes are inestimable. Use cuts simply like standard diet. It makes tasty virus sandwiches, French toast, garlic diet, and plunging diet. You can utilize it as a cheeseburger bun, make avocado toast bested with a poached egg, or truly anything you would do with customary diet.

What Makes This Keto Diet So Healthy?

If you've at any point taken a stab at preparing diet utilizing collagen protein as your primary "flour" source, then you realize that it is so testing to get it to remain cushioned and diet-like. My objective with this formula was to make a collagen-based keto diet that was as near standard diet as could reasonably be expected, with very low carbs and no dairy. This keto diet formula feels like I'm eating normal diet again and that can be useful, particularly when you're changing to a keto or Bulletproof diet.

Surprisingly better, this portion is standard size (not scaled down) and makes 12 liberal cuts. The macros per cut are around 77 calories, 5 grams of fat, 7 grams of protein, and 0 grams of net carbs (1 gram of carbs short 1 gram of fiber). You can without much of a stretch up the fat substance when expending this diet basically by slathering with grass-sustained ghee or margarine.

Add this keto diet formula to your armory of other great diet recipes that are paleo, keto and additionally Bulletproof. I think you'll think that its a great expansion to your formula box, and without a doubt when you're going ultra-low carb, this formula should ascend to the highest priority on your rundown.

BACON, EGG AND CHEESE CHAFFLE

We just got a smaller than expected waffle creator and it has become an immense hit in our home! We have utilized it around multiple times in the previous 3 days! We have been making Keto Chaffles which are fundamentally egg and cheddar and whatever else you need to blend in.

We have made treats, flame broiled cheddar sandwiches, Belgium waffles, and that's only the tip of the iceberg. My children even love utilizing it and are having some good times thinking of new things to make with it.

We are additionally attempting to eat less sugar and flour so making these bacon, egg, and cheddar chaffles have been ideal for the morning surge. Everyone takes about 2:30 minutes to make.

I don't care for the surface of fried eggs, however I love the delightful way these have somewhat fresh to them and are truly filling and brimming with season.

Recently I made an Everything Bagel Spice Chaffle and it was astonishing!! Today I had some remaining bacon in the ice chest that I chose to utilize.

They were so great and I think I have to twofold or triple the bunch so I can have more when I get eager!

They are so natural – blend the fixings, add them to the waffle producer, cook for 2:30 and it's finished!

This recipe makes 4 chaffles. You can place them in the ice chest and microwave them when you are ravenous.

I may likewise attempt to stick them into the toaster to perceive how they taste warmed.

Snap here to print the recipe for Keto bacon, egg, and cheddar Chaffles.

Keto Bacon, Egg, and Cheese Chaffles
2 eggs
3/4 cup cheddar
2 cuts cooked bacon
Guidelines:
Preheat your scaled down waffle creator. Splash with cooking oil.
Include the eggs and scramble them. Then include different fixings and blend well.
Pour 2 storing tablespoons of the hitter into the smaller than normal waffle creator.
Set a clock for 2:30 and pause.
When the time is done evacuate it with a fork. It will fresh us while you let it chill.
Discretionary – you can sprinkle some cheddar on to the egg blend before you close the waffle producer if you like additional cheddar season. It should give you that fresh cheddar enhance if you like that.
This chaffle breakfast sandwich meets up in under 10 minutes and makes eating keto or low carb diet a breeze! Just 3 Net Carbs for the entire sandwich!

The chaffle fever is as yet going solid and I love to think of different recipes that are fun and make the low carb or keto lifestyle a breeze! Breakfast sandwiches rush to make with chaffles because while the chaffle is cooking in your waffle iron, you can cook your egg in a skillet. Bacon or wiener patties can be cooked in the microwave so this entire whole breakfast sandwich meets up in less than 5 minutes. Judge me all you need yet that is the way I cook my bacon or wiener patties.

A chaffle is a waffle made of cheddar and an egg. It is essentially a play on consolidated words. There are various recipes for chaffles and some call for almond flour. I truly like the flavor of almond flour and that is the reason I add almond flour to my chaffles. A few people are hardcore chaffle fans and believe that a chaffle should just be an egg and cheddar. That is close to home inclination and one time somebody gave my chaffle recipe a low evaluating because of that. Entirely moronic as I would like to think however whatever I presume?

WHAT TYPE OF WAFFLE IRON SHOULD I USE?

I don't have a small scale waffle creator which is the thing that individuals are utilizing to make their chaffle buns or chaffle bread. I don't think a smaller than expected waffle iron is essential, however the scaled down waffles are pretty darn charming. I utilize my Villa waffle producer and afterward cut the chaffle down the middle to make a sandwich.

Run Mini Waffle Maker

Presto Ceramic FlipSide Waffle Maker

WHAT KIND OF CHEESE DO I NEED TO MAKE A CHAFFLE?

Mozzarella or cheddar are the two cheeses that are well known to make chaffles with. I've seen individuals use Monterey jack. Pepper jack cheddar would be great if you like zesty chaffles.

Step by step instructions to MAKE A CHAFFLE BREAKFAST SANDWICH

Preheat your waffle iron.

While the waffle iron is preheating, combine the cheddar, egg, and almond flour together in a bowl.

Shower the waffle iron with Cooking Spray and spread the hitter on to the waffle iron. Close it and let the waffle cook.

While the waffle is cooking cook your egg in a skillet. Make whatever kind of egg you like. Cook bacon in microwave.

Collect your chaffle breakfast sandwich and appreciate.

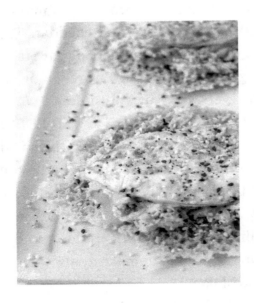

FANCY ROSEMARY AND GOAT CHEESE PANINI

I experienced childhood with sandwiches; was raised on them, truth be told. My dark colored sack lunch, alongside a hard-bubbled egg and a creased pack of Fritos, constantly included one of the accompanying top choices: bologna and mayonnaise, fish serving of mixed greens and lettuce, nutty spread and two cuts of American cheddar, cream cheddar and pepperoni. These odd sandwiches, consistently on white bread, were little and level — and never contenders for lunch swapping. (I additionally adored egg plate of mixed greens, however even as an eight-year-old realized that bubbled egg yolks and mayonnaise putrefying in a coat storage room for a large portion of a day is a perilous move, socially.)

Be that as it may, my preferred sandwich never made it to class. It was one cut of Wonder bread, deliberately spread with a layer of Philadelphia cream cheddar and beat with Smuckers purple jam. The bread was then collapsed fifty-fifty like a taco and eaten while sitting on our scratchy plaid couch, Elvis cover over my knees, watching a recurrent scene of Little House on the Prairie.

This recipe is a riff on that after-school treat. We've supplanted the cream cheddar with new chèvre from Dirty Girl Farm in Andes and the Smuckers with Westwind Orchard's raspberry jam, yet it's still sweet and appetizing and makes for a terrific breakfast, lunch, or treat. Matched with a jug of shimmering white wine* and an off the cuff outing at Thorn Preserve, it's a balance of youth sentimentality and adult refinement.

*Hild Elbling is our preferred at the present time. It's lemony, scandalous, invigorating and, as its merchant claims, "sufficiently light to drink a whole container and still work overwhelming hardware."

Fixings 6 Servings

4 ounces goat cheddar, chèvre, softened

2 tablespoons milk

2 tablespoons McCormick Gourmet™ Organic Basil

2 teaspoons McCormick Gourmet™ Organic Rosemary, Crushed

1 teaspoon McCormick Gourmet™ Organic Garlic Powder

1 teaspoon McCormick Gourmet™ Organic Thyme

1 teaspoon McCormick Gourmet™ Sicilian Sea Salt

2 infant eggplant, cut longwise in 1/4-inch thick cuts

2 medium portobello mushrooms, cut in 1/2-inch thick cuts

1 medium fennel bulb, cut and cut the long way in 1/4-inch thick cuts

1 chayote, cut in 1/4-inch thick cuts Substitutions accessible

1 red ringer pepper, cut in 2-inch strips

1 little red onion, cut into 1/2-inch thick adjusts

1/3 cup olive oil

Crisply ground McCormick Gourmet™ Organic Black Peppercorns, Whole

1 portion Ciabatta bread, split down the middle on a level plane

1 cup arugula leaves, washed and depleted.

Directions

18

Blend goat cheddar, milk, basil, rosemary, garlic powder, thyme and 1/2 teaspoon of the ocean salt in medium bowl until all around mixed. Put in a safe spot. Delicately brush vegetables with oil. Season with staying 1/2 teaspoon ocean salt and pepper

Flame broil over medium-high warmth 5 to 10 minutes or until vegetables are delicate, turning once. Expel vegetables from flame broil and keep warm. Barbecue bread parts 30 seconds for every side or until gently toasted

Spread goat cheddar blend equitably over each bread half. Layer 1/2 of the arugula, flame broiled vegetables and remaining arugula on 1 bread half. Top with second bread half. Cut sandwich into 1/2-inch wide segments to serve.

CARLIC BRAD CHAFFLE

If you're in the mind-set for some keto-accommodating mushy bread, this keto chaffle recipe is actually what you're searching for.

You can dunk it in marinara sauce, use it instead of a low-carb bread recipe, make a keto pizza out of it, or simply appreciate them as it stands.

Don't hesitate to stir up the cheddar also, cheddar and parmesan work extraordinary. What's more, if you truly need to go for the garlicky flavor, you can top it with some garlic spread.

These low-carb garlic bread chaffles are:

Exquisite

Delightful

Firm

Tasty

garlic cheddar bread chaffles

The primary fixings are:

Immaculate Keto Unflavored Whey Protein

Egg

Almond flour

garlic cheddar bread chaffles

garlic cheddar bread chaffles

Discretionary extra fixings

Parmesan cheddar

Mozzarella cheddar

Coconut flour

garlic cheddar bread chaffles

3 Health Benefits of Garlic Cheese Bread Chaffles

garlic cheddar bread chaffles

#1: Promotes Weight Loss

If you will likely shed some weight, then getting enough protein is fundamental. This simple keto chaffle recipe evades carbs and handled fixings, yet it's wealthy in protein also.

Protein is the most satisfying macronutrient when contrasted with carbs and fat. In any case, whey protein, specifically, has been appeared to lessen craving by expanding a feeling of fulfillment and deferring the arrival of your appetite.

One examination found that contrasted with casein and a glucose control, whey protein significantly affected satiety and completion in overweight individuals.

#2: Supports Heart Health

With cardiovascular illness taking the main space for the main source of death in the U.S., it's no big surprise that heart health is top of psyche for such a large number of individuals.

Markers for coronary illness incorporate high blood lipids, aggravation, oxidation stress, and obviously — blood pressure.

While there are a lot of pharmaceuticals out there that are intended to battle these hazard factors, the appropriate response might be covering up in your kitchen wash room.

Garlic has been utilized for a huge number of years as a recuperating plant. Research shows that enhancing with garlic concentrate can decrease hypertension (pulse), and furthermore check oxidative pressure, accordingly offering cardioprotection to individuals with high blood pressure.

#3: Protects Your Cell Membranes

Almonds are a superb wellspring of nutrient E, a fat-dissolvable nutrient. Nutrient E assumes various jobs in your body however has an especially basic job in the security of your cells.

Each phone in your body is secured by a layer of fat, called the lipid bilayer. Nutrient E, with its fondness for fat, goes about as a cancer prevention agent and ensures this lipid bilayer.

The harming impacts of free radicals on your cells can add to a wide scope of issues, including cardiovascular ailment and malignant growth. Therefore, ensuring your phone films by getting enough nutrient E through your eating routine is imperative for prevention.

This mushy garlic bread chaffle is the ideal supplement to your preferred Italian dinners. You can serve it before as a little canapé, or make it part of the principle dish.

Not at all like most breadsticks and rolls that commonly go with your dinners, this flavorful chaffle is sans gluten and works flawlessly into your keto diet feast plan.

We simply made the BEST Cheesy Garlic Bread Chaffle Recipe ever! If you need a straightforward canapé that presents truly quick, make this recipe! It will even be appreciated by your non-keto companions! Truly, they will adore it as well!

The keto diet has been so great to me. It's stunning keto chaffle recipes like this that keep things intriguing. It scarcely feels like whatever ought to be known as an eating routine. It's a lifestyle... it is for me in any case. I don't figure I would have said that the initial 4 months into my voyage however... I recall strikingly that it was so difficult to begin and kick the sugar and carbs addictions I used to confront.

Gooey GARLIC BREAD CHAFFLE RECIPE INGREDIENTS
(makes 2 gooey garlic bread chaffles)
Garlic Bread Chaffle Ingredients
1/2 cup mozzarella cheddar, destroyed

1 egg

1 tsp Italian flavoring

1/2 tsp garlic powder

1 tsp cream cheddar (I like to utilize seasoned cream cheddar, for example, chive and onion or jalapeno yet you can utilize plain as well)

Garlic Butter Topping Ingredients

1 tbs margarine

1/2 tsp Italian flavoring

1/2 tsp garlic powder

Mushy Bread Topping

2 tbs mozzarella cheddar, destroyed

run of parsley (or increasingly Italian flavoring)

Gooey GARLIC BREAD CHAFFLE RECIPE INSTRUCTIONS

Preheat your smaller than usual waffle producer.

Preheat your stove to 350F.

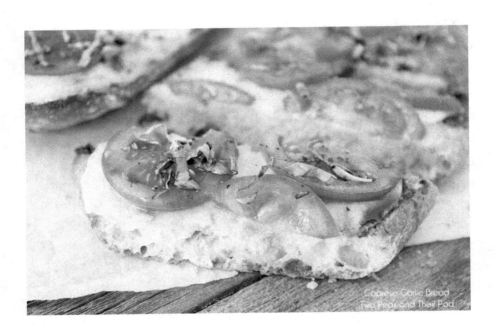

Caprese Garlic Bread
Two Peas and Their Pod

BAKED POTATO LOW CARB CHAFFLE

Heavenly Moly! This Baked Potato Chaffle is AMAZING! If you miss potatoes on the Keto diet, you are going to cherish this Keto chaffle recipe!

Heavenly Moly! This Jicama Loaded Baked Potato Chaffle is AMAZING! If you miss potatoes on the Keto diet, you are going to cherish this Keto chaffle recipe! Gigantic because of Cheryl W. from the Keto Chaffle Recipes Group for imparting these astounding recipes to us!

BAKED POTATO CHAFFLE RECIPE INGREDIENTS

1 enormous jicama root

1/2 medium onion, minced

2 garlic cloves, squeezed

1 cup cheddar of decision (I utilized Halloumi)

2 eggs, whisked

Salt and Pepper

Heated POTATO CHAFFLE RECIPE INSTRUCTIONS

Strip jicama and shred in nourishment processor

Spot destroyed jicama in an enormous colander, sprinkle with 1-2 tsp of salt. Blend well and permit to deplete.

Press out however much fluid as could reasonably be expected (significant advance)

Microwave for 5-8 minutes

Combine all fixings

Sprinkle a little cheddar on waffle iron before including 3 T of the blend, sprinkle somewhat more cheddar over the blend

Cook for 5 minutes. Flip and cook 2 more.

Top with a bit of harsh cream, bacon pieces, cheddar, and chives!

What is a jicama?

Jicama root is a round root vegetable local to Mexico that has a surface like a potato. It's low in calories and high in indispensable supplements. Jicama has around 5 net carbs per 100g. Jicama is stacked with fiber, nutrient c, and potassium! It additionally contains insoluble fiber.

If you haven't encountered jicama in your feasting collection, you have everything to pick up — and if you're wanting to shed some overabundance pounds, this may be your new top pick.

SUGAR COOKIE CHAFFLES

WOWZERS! Take a gander at this Chocolate Chip Cookie Chaffle Cake Recipe!! This is another Cheryl mixture of chaffle yet she utilized the chocolate chip treat recipe found in the Keto Friendly Recipes cookbook!!! How cool is that?!! There are huge amounts of recipes in that cookbook that can be made in the waffle producer. Actually, the chaffle recipe base fixings are the same old thing. Keto individuals have been making a cheddar based bread for quite a while now. Go to page 30 of that book and you will see the Jalapeno Cheese Bread recipe that uses the base recipe fixings that are precisely the same as the base for the fundamental chaffle recipe fixings.

In any case, this Chocolate Chip Cookie Chaffle Cake Recipe is astounding! This IS the thing that Low Carb dreams are made of! Keto dreams that is!

Update: This recipe made it to this rundown of BEST Chaffle Recipes on the web! If you love chaffles, you will see that rundown as overly accommodating!

Elements for cake layers:

1 tablespoon spread, dissolved

1 tablespoon Golden Monkfruit sugar

1 egg yolk

1/8 teaspoon vanilla concentrate

1/8 teaspoon cake player remove

3 tablespoons almond flour

1/8 teaspoon heating powder

1 tablespoon chocolate chips, sugar free

Whipped Cream Frosting Ingredients:

1 teaspoon unflavored gelatin

---

4 teaspoon cold water

1 cup substantial whipping cream

2 tablespoons confectioners' sugar

WHY IS IT CALLED A CHAFFLE?

It's known as a chaffle because cheddar + waffles = Chaffles! It's only a shrewd name that somebody in the keto network designed. Truly adorable, huh?!!

WHAT KITCHEN GADGET DO YOU USE TO MAKE CHAFFLES?

I love my little Mini Waffle Maker and I use it constantly. You can utilize a full-size waffle creator, simply be certain you twofold the recipe much of the time.

Would you be able to FREEZE CHAFFLES?

Truly, they hold up well! Simply make certain to wrap them firmly in a sealed shut holder to keep them new more. You can freeze them for as long as a month. I haven't tried any more extended than that.

Would you be able to MAKE CHAFFLES FOR A WHOLE WEEK AT ONE TIME?

You can likewise prepare early and make new chaffles for the week. They will remain new as long as you keep them refrigerated. To warm them, basically pop them in the microwave or air fryer to warm them up. The air fryer will in general get them pleasant and firm if that is the thing that you are going for!

This Pumpkin Chaffle Keto Sugar Cookies Recipe is ideal for fall. Sweet, chewy and delicate, these keto sugar treats have everything!

This Pumpkin Chaffle Keto Sugar Cookies Recipe is ideal for fall. Sweet, chewy and delicate, these keto sugar treats have everything!

Keto Chaffle Recipe eBook Cookbook

Keto Chaffle Recipes digital book

Keto Chaffle Recipes digital book

Searching FOR KETO CHAFFLE RECIPES? HERE YA GO!!!!

We have all the best keto chaffle recipes with new recipes being made day by day! In our new, Keto Chaffle Recipes eBook Cookbook, you will get over 50+ sweet and exquisite keto recipes for each flavor palette.

Essential Chaffle Recipes

Appetizing Chaffle Recipes

Sweet Chaffle Recipes

Chaffle Cake Recipes

CHOCOLATE CHIP COOKIE CHAFFLE

CHOCOLATE CHIP CHAFFLES are the least difficult contort on the most recent low carb furor, yet those small amounts of chocolate covering up all through the waffle are mystical. We serve our own with a major touch of whipped cream, however some low carb frozen yogurt would be a scrumptious garnish for dessert!

Keto Chocolate Chip Waffles! Only 3 net carbs per serving! #lowcarb #keto #chaffles #waffles

Indeed, it's legitimate.

Varieties to this recipe:

Include a tsp of cream cheddar to the player for included flavor Swap out coconut flour for almond flour. Coconut flour and almond flour are not a 1:1 substitution. By and large, the substitution is 1 section coconut flour to 4 sections almond flour, yet I have perused that in this recipe it is nearer to 1:3.

Swerve can be utilized rather than Lakanto Monkfruit, and the estimation is the equivalent.

More Chaffle Keto Recipes:

Profoundly Popular Traditional Keto Chaffle Recipe

The Very Best Pizza Chaffle Recipe

Maple Pumpkin Chaffle Keto Recipe

Taco Chaffle Recipe

Blueberry Keto Chaffle with almond flour

Little Keto Pizza with Chaffle Pizza Crust

Keto Chaffle Breakfast Sandwich with almond flour

The most effective method to Make Chocolate Chip Chaffle Keto Recipe:

Keto Chocolate Chip Chaffle Keto Recipe

This heavenly keto Chocolat Chip Chaffle Dessert Recipe is anything but difficult to make and tastes delightful. You can prepare a bunch in minutes to appreciate.

Planning Time

5 mins

Cook Time

8 mins

Course: bread, Breakfast, Dessert

Food: American, easygoing

Watchword: chaffle dessert, chaffle keto recipe, chocolate chip chaffle

Servings: 1Calories: 146kcalAuthor: Kasey Trenum

Fixings

1 egg

1 tbsp overwhelming whipping cream

1/2 tsp coconut flour

1 3/4 tsp Lakanto monkfruit brilliant can utilize pretty much to alter sweetness

1/4 tsp preparing powder

touch of salt

1 tbsp Lily's Chocolate Chips

Directions

Turn on the waffle creator with the goal that it warms up.

In a little bowl, consolidate all fixings with the exception of the chocolate chips and mix well until joined.

Oil waffle creator, then pour half of the hitter onto the base plate of the waffle producer. Sprinkle a couple of chocolate chips on top and afterward close.

Cook for 3-4 minutes or until the chocolate chip chaffle pastry is brilliant darker then expel from waffle producer with a fork, being mindful so as not to consume your fingers.

Rehash with the remainder of the hitter.

Let chaffle sit for a couple of moments so it starts to fresh. If wanted present with without sugar whipped besting.

Notes

The sugar alcohols from the Lakanto Monkfruit Golden are excluded from the healthful data since most subtract to figure net carbs.

Nourishment

Serving: 1g | Calories: 146kcal | Carbohydrates: 7g | Protein: 6g | Fat: 10g | Saturated Fat: 7g | Fiber: 3g | Sugar: 1g

GINGERBREAD

An immortal, exemplary, conventional Gingerbread recipe! This is one of my family's preferred recipes. It makes for a thick however delicate, clammy, and luxuriously seasoned gingerbread, impeccably enhanced with molasses, dark colored sugar, and heaps of comfortable flavors!

Appreciate!

MORE RECIPES YOU MAY ENJOY:

Gingerbread Cupcakes

Molasses Cookies

Gingerbread Fudge

Gingerbread Layer Cake

The most effective method to MAKE GINGERBREAD

Make certain to look at my Gingerbread Recipe VIDEO just underneath the recipe! If you appreciate these recordings, if it's not too much trouble consider buying in to my YouTube Channel so you can be the first to see the entirety of my cooking recordings

Gingerbread

An exemplary gingerbread recipe! Firmly adjusted from Good Housekeeping (offshoot).

4.88 from 31 votes

Print Pin Rate

Course: DessertCuisine: AmericanKeyword: christmas recipe, gingerbread, occasion heating, recipe with molassesPrep Time: 20 minutesCook Time: 45 minutesTotal Time: 1 hour 5 minutesServings: 9 enormous slicesCalories: 400kcalAuthor: Sam Merritt

Fixings

33

½ cup unsalted margarine (ideally European spread) softened to room temperature (113g)

½ cup dim darker sugar firmly stuffed (100g)

1 cup unsulphured molasses (235ml) (I utilize Grandma's image)

1 huge egg

1 teaspoon vanilla concentrate

2 ½ cups generally useful flour (312g)

1 ½ teaspoon preparing pop

1 teaspoon ground cinnamon

1 teaspoon ground ginger

½ teaspoon ground cloves

¾ teaspoon salt

1 cup bubbling water (235ml)

Whipped Cream for fixing, discretionary

Guidelines

Preheat broiler to 350F (175C) and set up a 9"x9" preparing dish by either liberally lubing and flouring or by fixing with material paper. Put in a safe spot.

Join spread and dark colored sugar in an enormous bowl and utilize an electric blender to beat until velvety.

Include molasses and mix until very much consolidated.

Include egg and vanilla concentrate. Mix well.

In a different bowl, whisk together flour, preparing pop, ground cinnamon, ground ginger, ground cloves, and salt.

Step by step add dry fixings to wet until totally consolidated.

Cautiously mix in bubbling water until fixings are smooth and well-consolidated.

Empty hitter into arranged preparing container and heat on 350F (175C) for 40 minutes or until a toothpick embedded in the inside tells the truth or with a couple of clammy scraps.

Permit to cool before cutting and serving. This Gingerbread tastes best when topped with whipped cream!

The most effective method to make gingerbread bread rolls:

Include spread, brilliant syrup and light dark colored sugar to a dish. Mix on a low warmth until sugar has broken up.

Include flour, bicarbonate of pop and ginger to a combining bowl then mix. Make a well in the middle and pour in the sugar and margarine blend.

Mix together to frame a mixture (it may be most effortless to utilize your hands).

Enclose by clingfilm and let chill for 30mins to solidify.

Lay the batter between two sheets of heating material. Press mixture delicately with a moving pin. Give a quarter turn than rehash.

Give it a last quarter turn, then begin to move in reverse and advances, giving ordinary quarter turns. Until batter is generally thickness of a £1 coin.

Utilizing a scone shaper cut out the shapes. Heat at 190°C (170°C fan) mark 5 for 10 to 12min, until gently brilliant dark colored.

The bread rolls won't be firm however will solidify when left to cool outside the broiler.

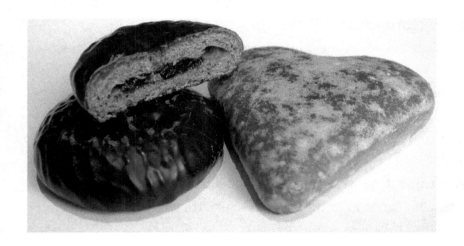

BOSTOM CREAM PIE CHAFFLE

Fixings

Chaffle Cake Ingredients:

2 eggs

1/4 cup almond flour

1 tsp coconut flour

2 tbsp liquefied spread

2 tbsp cream cheddar room temp

20 drops Boston Cream remove

1/2 tsp vanilla concentrate

1/2 tsp heating powder

2 tbsp swerve confectioners' sugar or monkfruit

1/4 tsp Xanthan powder

Custard Ingredients:

1/2 cup substantial whipping cream

1/2 tsp Vanilla concentrate

1/2 tbs Swerve confectioners Sweetener

2 Egg Yolks

1/8 tsp Xanthan Gum

Ganache Ingredients:

2 tbs substantial whipping cream

2 tbs Unsweetened Baking chocolate bar slashed

1 tbs Swerve Confectioners Sweetener

Boston Cream Pie gets a keto makeover! I as of late refreshed this low carb formula and now it's shockingly better than previously, with less carbs. Delicate almond flour cake loaded up with sugar free vanilla cake cream and a rich low carb chocolate coat.

Keto Boston Cream Pie formula - a cut of the cake on white plate with raspberries, with the remainder of the cake on a white cake remain out of sight

BANANA NUT CHAFFLES

I simply made the BEST Banana Nut Chaffle Recipe I've at any point attempted! Omgosh, It's stunning!

Here's the mystery fixing however... You can't do bananas on the keto diet. They are truly elevated carb so you need to stay away from them however much as could be expected. In the event that you love the flavor of banana, you completely should get some banana remove! It's a distinct advantage! I utilize the Lorann Banana Extract here. There are huge amounts of great banana separate brands you can get. Here are a couple of we would prescribe:

Next, you completely need a small waffle creator! Run makes the best! Presently, you needn't bother with the scaled down however you do require a waffle creator. In the event that you have a full-size waffle producer, you can totally utilize that however simply ensure you twofold the formula!

BANANA NUT CHAFFLE RECIPE INGREDIENTS

1 egg

1 tbs cream cheddar. relaxed and room temp

1 tbs sugar free cheesecake pudding (discretionary fixing since it is messy keto)

1/2 cup mozzarella cheddar

1 tbs Monkfruit confectioners

1/4 tsp vanilla concentrate

1/4 tsp banana remove

Discretionary Toppings:

Sugar free caramel sauce (we have a natively constructed caramel sauce form here: How to Make Sugar Free Caramel Sauce)

Walnuts (or any of your preferred nuts)

BANANA NUT CHAFFLE RECIPE INSTRUCTIONS

Preheat the small scale waffle creator

In a little bowl, whip the egg.

Add the rest of the fixings to the egg blend and blend it until it's very much fused.

Add a large portion of the player to the waffle creator and cook it for at least 4 minutes until it's brilliant darker.

Evacuate the completed chaffle and include the other portion of the hitter to cook the other chaffle.

Fixings:

1/2 cup of cheddar, destroyed (you can utilize any cheddar)

1 egg

1 tsp of sans gluten preparing powder

2 tablespoons of almond flour (can substitute with 1 tablespoon of coconut flour whenever wanted)

Guidelines:

Assemble and set up the entirety of your fixings and preheat your waffle creator.

Combine your egg, destroyed cheddar, heating powder, and almond or coconut flour.

Empty a large portion of your blend into the waffle producer. Cook till done. Expel. Empty the rest of the hitter into the waffle creator and cook.

We purchased the little Dash brand smaller than normal waffle creator and the scaled down frying pan (you can utilize it is possible that one) to use with this formula and it makes the ideal size Chaffle. Try not to have a small scale waffle creator? You can utilize a normal waffle producer or skillet after all other options have been exhausted.

Chaffle Variations

For every variety, you will consolidate the fixings recorded at that point cook similarly as you would the essential Chaffle formula. When cooking chaffle just add roughly 2 to 2 1/2 tablespoons of player to the smaller than normal waffle producer. In the event that you are utilizing a customary size waffle producer split the hitter down the middle.

These varieties make 3 to 4 servings.

Bacon Chaffle

1 egg

1/2 cup cheddar, destroyed

2 Tbsp almond flour

1 tsp heating powder

3 Tbsp cooked bacon disintegrates

Blueberry Muffin Chaffle

1/2 cup of mozzarella cheddar, destroyed

1 egg

1 tsp of heating powder

2 tablespoons of almond flour

2 tsp of sugar

Bunch of blueberries

2 tablespoon of slashed nuts (discretionary)

Blueberry Muffin Chaffle

Cinnamon Roll Chaffle

1/2 cup of mozzarella cheddar, destroyed

1 egg

1 tsp of heating powder

2 tablespoons of almond flour

1 to 2 tsp of cinnamon

1 tsp of vanilla

1 tsp of sugar

Nut Butter Chaffle

1 egg

1/2 cup mozzarella cheddar

1 tsp vanilla

1 tablespoon sugar

2 Tbsp nut margarine

1/2 tsp of heating powder

2 tablespoons of almond flour

Top with natively constructed whipping cream for a treat.

Lemon Delight Chaffle

1 oz cream cheddar (relaxed)

1/4 cup mozzarella cheddar, destroyed

1 egg

1 to 2 tsp lemon juice

2 tablespoons of sugar

1 tsp heating powder

4 tablespoons of almond flour

This is extraordinary with some cream cheddar icing.

Banana Nut Muffin Chaffle

1 oz cream cheddar (mellowed)

1/4 cup mozzarella cheddar, destroyed

1 egg

1 tsp banana remove

2 tablespoons of sugar

1 tsp preparing powder

4 tablespoons of almond flour

2 tablespoons of pecans or walnuts, cleaved

Pizza Chaffle

1 egg

1/2 cup cheddar, destroyed

1 Tbsp keto inviting marinara sauce

2 Tbsp pepperoni (cut into little pieces)

1 tsp of preparing powder

4 tablespoon almond flour

1 tsp of Italian flavoring

These are incredible topped with parmesan cheddar.

Oreo Chaffle

1 egg

1/2 cup of mozzarella cheddar, destroyed

1/2 tsp of preparing powder

2 tablespoons of cacao powder

2 tablespoons of sugar

2 tablespoon of almond flour

These are incredible topped with cream cheddar icing.

McGriddle Chaffle

1 egg

1 oz cream cheddar, mollified

1 tsp sugar

1 tsp vanilla

1 tablespoon keto-accommodating maple syrup (We use Lakanto)
1/4 cup mozzarella cheddar, destroyed
1 tsp of preparing powder
4 tablespoons of almond flour

Chocolate Dream Chaffle

1 egg
1/4 cup of mozzarella cheddar
1 oz cream cheddar
2 tsp sugar
2 tablespoons cacao powder
1 tsp vanilla
4 Tbsp almond flour
1 tsp preparing powder
Red Velvet Chaffle
1 egg
1/4 cup of mozzarella cheddar
1 oz cream cheddar
2 tsp sugar
2 tablespoons cacao powder
1 tsp red velvet concentrate
4 Tbsp almond flour
1 tsp heating powder
This is so great with some cream cheddar icing.

ChaffleTortillas

1 egg
1/2 cup cheddar, destroyed
4 tablespoon of almond flour

1 tsp heating powder

1/2 to 1 tablespoon of almond milk or substantial whipping cream

1/4 tsp of garlic powder

We make these in a skillet rather than the waffle creator with the goal that we can get them looking like a tortilla.

Macros:

Fundamental Chaffle Recipe

Serving Size: 1 serving (2 Chaffles)

Supplement

Calories

Net Carbs

Fiber

Protein

Fat

All out Carbs Value

380

2.0 g

2.0 g

22 g

31 g

5.0 g

CARROT CAKE CHAFFLE

Basic exemplary flavor in a waffle cake structure total with delicious cream cheddar icing. This is my life partner's most mentioned cake and now he can have it low carb!

? I'm not going to mislead anybody, I licked the bowl! ?

CARROT CHAFFLE CAKE RECIPE INGREDIENTS

Carrot Chaffle Cake fixings

1/2 cup carrot, destroyed

1 egg

2 T spread, liquefied

2 T overwhelming whipping cream

3/4 cup almond flour

1 T pecans, cleaved

2 T powdered sugar

2 tsp cinnamon

1 tsp pumpkin flavor

1 tsp preparing powder

Cream Cheese Frosting

4 oz cream cheddar, mellowed

1/4 cup powdered sugar

1 tsp vanilla concentrate

1-2 T substantial whipping cream (contingent upon the consistency you like)

CARROT CHAFFLE CAKE RECIPE INSTRUCTIONS

Blend your dry fixings – almond flour, cinnamon, pumpkin zest, heating powder, powdered sugar, and pecan pieces.

Include the wet fixings ground carrot, egg, dissolved spread, overwhelming cream.

Add 3 T hitter to preheated small waffle creator. Cook 2 1/2 – 3 minutes.

Combine icing fixings with a hand blender with whisk connection until all around consolidated.

Stack waffles and include icing between each layer!

CARROT CHAFFLE CAKE RECIPE NUTRITION INFORMATION

Makes 6 Chaffles. (Servings) 2.4 net carbs without icing. 3.7 net carbs with icing. 1/4 of cake is 5.5 net carbs!

STRAWBERRY SHORTCAKE CHAFFLE

I simply made the most brilliant Strawberry Shortcake Chaffle Recipe! OMGosh, you must attempt it! The introduction for this sweet keto-accommodating pastry was additional uncommon as well! We acquired these charming minimal individual size cake plates only for these pastry chaffles! Did you see the charming Pumpkin Cake Chaffle Recipe we posted not long ago! It's gone insane viral and everybody is adoring that formula!

STRAWBERRY SHORTCAKE CHAFFLE RECIPE
INGREDIENTS

1 egg

1/4 cup mozzarella cheddar

1 tbs cream cheddar

1/4 tsp heating powder

2 strawberries, cut

1 tsp strawberry separate STRAWBERRY SHORTCAKE CHAFFLE RECIPE INSTRUCTIONS

Preheat waffle producer.

In a little bowl, whip the egg.

Include the rest of the fixings.

Shower the waffle producer with nonstick cooking splash.

Gap blend fifty-fifty.

Cook a large portion of the blend for around 4 minutes or until brilliant dark colored.

STRAWBERRY SHORTCAKE CHAFFLE RECIPE NUTRITION LABEL INFORMATION

(this does exclude the garnishes, just the chaffle) Makes 2 chaffles.

Discretionary Glaze: 1 tbs cream cheddar warmed in the microwave for 15 seconds, 1/4 tsp strawberry concentrate, and 1 tbs monkfruit confectioners mix.

Blend and spread over the warm waffle.

Discretionary Cream Cheese Frosting: 1 tbs cream cheddar (room temp), 1/4 tsp strawberry separate, 1 tbs room temp margarine (room temp), and 1 tbs monkfruit confectioners mix.

Combine all fixings and spread over the waffle.

You can likewise top it with basic whipped cream and strawberries.

Custom made whipped cream: 1 cup overwhelming whipping cream, 1 tsp vanilla, 1 tbs monkfruit confectioners mix. Whip until it structures tops. Simple peasy!

Strawberry Shortcake Chaffles. This low carb and keto benevolent Strawberry Shortcake Chaffle is the ideal sweet to appreciate after supper! A sweet chaffle beat with hand crafted keto whipped cream and sweet strawberries! On the off chance that you are searching for a keto strawberry shortcake or a low carb strawberry shortcake then this will before long become your go to!

Strawberry Shortcake Chaffle

Strawberry Shortcake Keto Chaffle Recipe

Strawberry Shortcake Keto Chaffle

This keto Strawberry Shortcake is the most up to date chaffle formula that I am adding to the chaffle plans here on the blog. Furthermore, similar to the next chaffle plans we have shared this one is absolutely delish!

One of my preferred sweets is Strawberry shortcake. I love the sweet kind of the strawberries, blended in with the sweetness of the cake and whipped cream. Anyway my preferred strawberry shortcake formula isn't low carb using any and all means so while adhering to low carb it has been a no go. At that point the keto chaffle formula detonated facebook and I realized I could transform that into a tasty low carb strawberry shortcake formula with a couple tweeks.

I will caution you however, when I was making it I didn't anticipate that it should be as stunning as it turned out. I expected to have a few similitudes, yet not to be great. Anyway the final product is thoroughly astonishing, absolutely great and I presently don't need to leave my strawberry shortcake dessert behind. I would now be able to appreciate it at whatever point I need to!

While this keto chaffle is sufficiently sweet to be a pastry, it is likewise ideal for a high fat low carb breakfast. That is correct, this generally a treat thing can be delighted in for breakfast with no blame by any stretch of the imagination!

What is a Chaffle?

Are every one of your companions discussing chaffles and you are attempting to make sense of what they are? It's alright , they are astonishing and you will cherish them. Be that as it may, just put a chaffle is a waffle made with egg and cheddar. Presently from the essential chaffle formula you can make MANY various assortments of chaffles simply switching up the sort of cheddar that you use.

You can likewise switch up the flavors by adding various things to the fundamental chaffle formula. There are truly unlimited conceivable outcomes when making keto chaffles.

On the off chance that you are new to making chaffles make certain to look at how to make a chaffle for the best keto chaffle formula. This is the place all chaffles, including this pastry chaffle formula start.

Keto Chocolate Chaffle

Blueberry Chaffle

Pizza Chaffle

Cinnamon Roll Chaffle

Chaffle Breakfast Sandwich

Is a Mini Waffle Maker required?

While I like to utilize my dah scaled down waffle producer, you can make this keto strawberry shortcake formula in a huge waffle creator. It will make 3 little chaffles or 1 huge keto chaffle.

Strawberry Shortcake Chaffles Ingredients

Strawberries

granulated swerve

Keto Whipped Cream

Almond flour

egg

mozzarella cheddar

vanilla concentrate

The most effective method to Make Strawberry Shortcake Chaffles

Course Breakfast

Planning Time 30 minutes

Cook Time 19 minutes

Rise Time 1 hour 10 minutes

Complete Time 1 hour 59 minutes

Servings 12

Calories 618kcal

Creator Julie Clark

Fixings

For the Dough:

1 cup warm milk (around 115 degrees F)

2 1/2 teaspoons moment dry yeast (I like Red Star Platinum Baking Yeast)

2 huge eggs at room temperature

1/3 cup spread softened

4 1/2 cups generally useful flour

1 teaspoon salt

1/2 cup granulated sugar

For the Filling:

1/2 cup spread nearly softened

1 cup stuffed darker sugar

2 tablespoons cinnamon

1/2 cup overwhelming cream (for pouring over the risen rolls)

For the Frosting:

6 ounces cream cheddar (mollified)

1/3 cup spread (relaxed)

2 cups powdered sugar

1/2 tablespoon maple concentrate (or vanilla)

Directions

Pour the warm milk in the bowl of a stand blender and sprinkle the yeast overtop.

Include the eggs, spread, salt and sugar.

Include the flour and blend utilizing the mixer edge just until the fixings are scarcely consolidated. Enable the blend to rest for 5 minutes so the flour has the opportunity to absorb the fluids.

Scratch the batter off the mixer edge and expel it. Join the mixture snare.

Beat the batter on medium speed for 5-7 minutes or until the mixture is flexible and smooth. **The batter will be shabby will at present be adhering to the sides of the bowl. That is alright! Try not to be enticed to include more flour now.

Shower an enormous bowl with cooking splash.

Utilize an elastic spatula to expel the mixture from the blender bowl and spot it in the lubed enormous bowl.

PECAN PIE CHAFFLE

This is a genuine festival from this Southern young lady to you all! I was brought up in the North GA mountains and have affectionate recollections of getting paper sacks brimming with walnuts from my grandparent's back yard. Breaking and shelling them wasn't an excessive amount of fun, yet I realized the prize would be a yummy, gooey, newly prepared walnut pie. I've taken all that flavor and pressed it into a Low Carb Chaffle Cake.

To begin with, I might want to make reference to that this formula is low carb in light of the backstrap molasses fixing. It assists with the shading and the flavor. You can get a lighter, more keto-accommodating formula by including a keto-accommodating syrup in as a trade for this fixing. I would utilize maple syrup from Lakanto or Jordan's thin syrup that has a comparable flavor.

Walnut Pie Filling Ingredients

2 tablespoons spread, mellowed

1 tablespoon Sukrin Gold

1/8 teaspoon blackstrap molasses, discretionary yet assists with shading and flavor

2 tablespoons Maple Bourbon Pecan Skinny Syrup

2 tablespoons overwhelming whipping cream

2 huge egg yolks

Squeeze salt

2 tablespoons walnuts, daintily toasted (I did it in the Airfryer)

Walnut Pie Chaffle Ingredients

1 egg

1 tablespoon overwhelming whipping cream

---

2 tablespoons cream cheddar, mellowed

1/2 teaspoon maple remove (Olive Nation)

3 tablespoons almond flour

1 tablespoon oat fiber (or another tablespoon almond flour)

1 tablespoon Sukrin Gold

1/2 teaspoon heating powder

2 tablespoons walnuts, slashed

Walnut PIE CHAFFLE CAKE FILLING INSTRUCTIONS

Include margarine, sugar, overwhelming whipping cream and syrups to a little pot on low warmth.

Rush until all around consolidated.

Expel from heat.

Pour 1/2 of the blend into egg yolks and whisk well.

Include that blend once again into the pot while mixing consistently.

Include a touch of salt and walnut.

Let stew until it begins to thicken.

Expel from warmth and let cool while making the Chaffles.

Walnut PIE CHAFFLE CAKE RECIPE INSTRUCTIONS

Blend all fixings aside from walnuts in a little blender for around 15 seconds.

Stop and scratch down the sides with a spatula, and keep blending for an additional 15 seconds until all around mixed.

Blend in walnuts with a spatula.

Pour 3 T of hitter in preheated small waffle creator.

Cook for 1/2 mins.

Expel to cooling rack.

Rehash.

Will make 3 full Chaffles with a modest one for tasting!

Put 1/3 of the walnut pie filling on each Chaffle and gather as wanted!

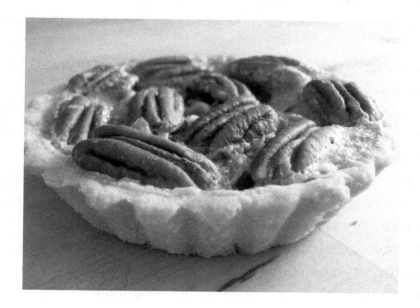

LEMON MERINGUE CHAFFLE

I am so amped up for this...

This lemon pie possesses a flavor like an eruption of Summertime moving over your tongue!

It takes somewhat longer than the plans that I generally present yet it's going on merit each ounce of exertion that you put into it.

As a matter of first importance, the outside layer is my new most loved low carb pie hull.

It consolidates the fresh sweetness of almond flour with the sandy surface of coconut flour. It's somewhat suggestive of shortbread in the most magnificent manner.

I believe it will need to turn into its very own formula so the entirety of my Keto companions can discover it and fill it with whatever they can consider.

Individuals on the Keto Diet will in general be super (ahem) inventive when searching for low carb dessert options.

Slanting Content from Castle in the Mountains Second, the lemony flavor will make you pucker up (positively).

I was wary about making this pie... lemon pie has consistently been a most loved warm climate treat around here and I was concerned that it would crash and burn against my desires.

In any case, it was fan-cracking tastic and adequate that I needed to share it (not all plans make the cut you know).

Pie Crust

(This post may contain offshoot joins. As an Amazon Associate I will make a little commission at no expense to you when you make a passing buy.)

Tips for a fabulous outside layer:

Ensure your spread is cold.

This is an unquestionable requirement for any pie outside layer, Keto or not. Leave it in the refrigerator until you are prepared to cut it up and hurl it in the nourishment processor.

I really utilize a Ninja blender. I have a nourishment processor yet its enormous and an agony to clean.

The blender accompanies distinctive measured "pitchers" for making an assortment of whatever it is you are making. All aspects of my blender other than the engine is dishwasher safe so... it wins inevitably.

Furthermore, it was extremely reasonable (another success).

Heartbeat the fixings until they are pea measured.

Try not to mix up the outside layer until its "uniform". You need a few bits of margarine in there making your outside flaky and light.

Press the batter into the pie skillet.

I utilized my knuckles and afterward the base of a glass to kind of even it out.

Press in pie coverings are one of my preferred advantages of making Keto pie outside layers... not any more revealing the mixture. It's never been one of my qualities.

Heat the hull and let it cool while you are making the pie filling. It ought to be cool when you finish.

Emptying the filling into a hot pie outside layer will make it spongy and you'll wind up eating your pie with a spoon.

Get together THE FILLING INGREDIENTS... .

lemon meringue pie fixings

It will be simpler on the off chance that you separate your eggs into yolks and whites and beat the yolks in a grain bowl or something comparative.

You'll require space to "temper" the eggs with the hot blend later all the while.

You'll be utilizing both egg whites and yolks in the event that you intend to make the meringue.

Lemon pizzazz is significant and it develops the kind of the filling.

The formula records 2-3 tablespoons of pizzazz. I zested every one of the four lemons and utilized anyway a lot of I had on the grounds that I love the harshness that it includes.

It's a "to taste" kind of fixing.

Ground cardamom is discretionary.

Yet, you should utilize it on the off chance that you have it. I can't depict the flavor aside from citrusy, and home grown.

Cardamom fabricates the pie's flavor in intricacy and whoever is sufficiently fortunate to impart it to you will be left thinking about what the mystery fixing is.

What to do in the event that you don't have psyllium husk powder...

Purchase some...just joking.

In any case, not so much, get some for some time later on the grounds that it destroys thickener.

I like psyllium husk powder due to the fiber and the surface. Be that as it may, I know not every person keeps it close by. Also, it's not in every case promptly accessible at a market (yet).

You can utilize 2 teaspoons of arrowroot powder if important. (Even my supermarket in the sticks has it).

I truly cant address how much thickener to utilize on the grounds that I don't utilize it any longer. I wager it would work... I simply cant help with the conversion scale.

Since I found how much simpler psyllium husk powder functions, tastes and the stunning medical advantages it has... I have been utilizing it only in my prepared products starting late. On the off chance that YOU WILL BE MAKING THE MERINGUE...

I truly like my Lemon Pie with whipped cream.

I have never been a tremendous devotee of meringue yet individuals like it. It keeps well in the cooler and ventures well (Whipped cream DOES NOT).

What's more, it looks excellent so I remembered meringue for this formula and even put it on BOTH of my Lemon Pies.

For what reason did I make two pies?

Since I "over beat" the meringue on the principal pie.

I beat the egg whites until they were frothy like a bowl loaded with dish washing fluid.

This is the thing that occurred... .

over beaten meringue

Do you see that emptied out arch of crunchy meringue like stuff?

That's right. It looked delightful outwardly however I was really frustrated with the last item.

Despite everything we ate it... however a crunchy and super-sweet garnish was not what I was going for.

It was alright in light of the fact that it was then that I understood it required more thickener... and I had the option to caution you about over beating the eggs.

(I have never had this occur and at first accused the erythritol lol.)

Side note:

Since I made two pies and attempted two pies and LOVE lemon pie, I went WAY over my cutoff of erythritol... and it was revolting.

While I won't (over)share precisely what occurred, I will let you know this..only eat each cut in turn.

Try not to OVERDO IT regardless of the amount you love lemon pie.

This formula calls for hardened tops for the meringue... not froth.

It should look something like this.

hardened crested meringue

Simply thud the egg whites over the filling and spread to the outside.

There is no smooth method to do this. On the off chance that you have never made meringue, don't stress.

You'll get the hang of spreading it out before long.

Which is great since you would prefer not to delay a lot now. Try not to let the meringue flatten a lot before you seal it up and get this infant in the broiler.

meringue on pie

Ensure the meringue seals the whole pie in.

I don't have a clue why you must be cautious about this, I simply realize you do.

My Gram resembled Wonder Woman in the kitchen and she repeated this point so a lot of that I have never attempted to make sense of what occurs on the off chance that you don't close it... .

Perhaps it spills out? Possibly it flattens? I don't have the foggiest idea yet you should simply pursue her recommendation and be cautious with this progression.

The pinnacles of the meringue ought to be a light brilliant dark colored.

Since the pie outside is fixed in you would truly need to prepare it for quite a while to consume it..but consumed meringue isn't great either.

Prepare for 30-35 minutes or until sautéed and it doesn't shake when you squirm the pie skillet.

THAT'S IT...

I trust you make the most of your lemon pie and please let me know in the remarks underneath in the event that you have any inquiries or very marvelous increases!

Compelling Keto Lemon Meringue Pie

Keto Lemon Merigue Pie

I LOVE LEMON PIE! It's invigorating and just poses a flavor like Summer. This is an incredible formula for an uncommon event or after a flavorful dinner. You can make this with or without the meringue. I would state this low carb treat takes a smidgen of kitchen abilities however anybody can pull it off in the event that you adhere to the directions.

3.5 from 6 votes

Print Pin Rate

Course: DessertCuisine: American, keto dessert, low carb dessertKeyword: keto dessert, keto lemon merigue pie, Low carb lemon merigue pie Prep Time: 30 minutesCook Time: 30 minutesCooling Time: 5 hoursTotal Time: 1 hour Servings: 8 Slices Calories: 294kcal Author: Brenna Ring

Fixings

Pie Crust

1/2 Cup Almond Flour

1/2 Cup Coconut Flour

2 Tbsp Erythritol

2 tsp Psyllium Husk powder

2 huge eggs

1/2 cup Butter (salted) cubed and VERY cold

Pie Filling

1 Cup Erythritol

1 bundle Unflavored Gelatin I utilized Knox

4 Egg Yolks beaten (save whites for meringue)

1 Cup Water

1 tbsp Psyllium Husk Powder

3 tbsp Salted Cream Butter

1 Cup Lemon Juice Fresh is ideal. I utilized four lemons.

2-3 tbsp Lemon Zest I zested each of the four lemons and utilized what I had. This is a "to taste" sort of fixing.

1 tsp ground cardamom discretionary

* Meringue

4 Egg Whites

1/2 tsp Cream of Tartar

1/8-1/4 cup low carb sugar *to taste (see notes in post)

US Customary - Metric

Get Ingredients Powered by Chicory

Guidelines

Pie Crust

Preheat broiler to 350F

Put everything into a blender or nourishment processor and heartbeat until it the consistency of pieces.

Press into a pie plate and heat for 10-12 minutes.

Significant: Let the outside layer cool totally before you fill it.

Pie Crust

Filling

Beat the egg yolks in a bowl and let sit until the subsequent stage is finished.

Join sugar, gelatin, psyllium husk powder, and water in a pan. Heat to the point of boiling for one moment while always mixing with a whisk.

Empty a portion of the blend into the bowl with the beaten eggs while mixing (this is called treating).

Empty the egg blend again into the pot and stew until thickened. Try not to allow this to bubble! IT HAS TO THICKEN IN THE PAN OR IT WILL STAY SOUPY. Prop stirring....it's up to look somewhat vile and unusual from the outset. This will level out in the following stage.

Race in the salted spread, lemon juice and lemon get-up-and-go. Expel from warmth and let cool for 20 minutes.

Immerse your pie covering and let cool to room temp or put it in the ice chest to speed it up.

In the event that you are including the meringue, move onto the subsequent stage.

On the off chance that you will be beating your pie with whipped cream, leave the pie in the ice chest until cold and you are prepared to serve.

Merigue

Let the pie filling cool for in any event 15 minutes at room temp or put it in the cooler for 10 minutes to speed this up.

* This is significant. It would be ideal if you see tips in the post.

Whip the egg whites, cream of tartar and sugar until hardened pinnacles frame yet don't over beat. *see tips in post

I utilize a Kitchen help for this progression however

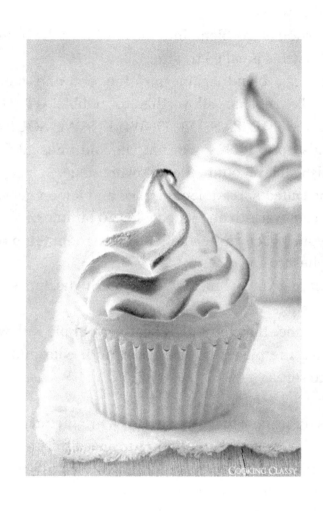

TACO CHAFFLES

This Crispy Taco Chaffle Recipe is completely mouth-watering flavorful! It was such an unbelievable expansion to the Very Best Taco Meat, and the firm taco shells were superior to anything I envisioned.

Taco Chaffle Recipe: Crispy, Not Eggy, and Delicious!

Taco servings of mixed greens are one of our preferred simple family dinners. Every one of the four children love tacos. They can make the most of theirs on tortillas, while the centers and I eat taco plates of mixed greens or here and there keto taco cups. I've taken a stab at making taco dishes simply out of cheddar, and despite the fact that I love the crunch, they are constantly somewhat oily.

At that point, enter all the Keto Chaffle absurdity that has set the keto world ablaze of late. As I was preparing supper the previous evening, I realized that I could make a Chaffle Taco Shell effectively. While there are numerous chaffle plans on the web, I realized that this one should have been incredibly firm and not eggy at all or it could never go as a taco shell.

My most established girl and I began testing and thought of without a doubt the ideal and firm taco shell chaffle. It was so great; I needed to make more since we adored it to such an extent. I've incorporated all the data you need underneath on the off chance that you aren't exactly cutting-edge on this chaffle insane.

Anyway, What in the World is a Chaffle?

I know. It has been a serious week in the keto network. On the off chance that you took some time off or haven't invested any energy in Facebook gatherings, you may have passed up the chaffle rage. A Chaffle is a waffle made on a Dash Mini Waffle Maker with eggs and cheddar. Since that formula turned out, there have been incalculable varieties posted, and some don't have any cheddar as a fixing. This formula for Keto Taco Chaffles is a variety of the first formula that I tried until I got an ideal firm taco shell chaffle. Make a point to look at this rundown of Ultimate Tips for Best Keto Chaffle Recipes.

What Do I Use to Make a Keto Taco Chaffle?

The Dash Mini Waffle Maker is the one kitchen machine that the keto world has been set for find. This smaller than usual waffle producer makes one four-inch waffle. While you could utilize a normal waffle producer, there is something in particular about this smaller than expected one that gets Chaffles pleasant and firm. Maybe it is on the grounds that the meshes are littler and closer together or the way that it gets so hot, however in any case, there is no uncertainty that on the off chance that you pursue the Keto Diet, you are going to see many plans for this item.

For the individuals who may feel that creation each chaffle in turn is excessively particular, this waffle creator is an extraordinary alternative. It makes four 3 inch waffles without a moment's delay. Since it makes littler Chaffles, you'd have to utilize somewhat less hitter, however it could be a tremendous timesaver on the off chance that you are making a few Keto Chaffle taco shells on the double.

Where Can I Find the Dash Mini Waffle Maker?

On the off chance that you would prefer not to go around town on a scrounger chase searching for a waffle creator in stores, you can put in a request on Amazon. The way that Amazon conveys without me hauling every one of my children around town implies that it is forever my first decision. In the event that you need to get one without requesting check Bed Bath and Beyond, TJ Maxx, Kohl's, Walmart, or Target.

To begin with, I began by tossing every one of the fixings in a little bowl. I utilized a blend of thicker destroyed cheddar for Taco Chaffles.

Daintily oil the Dash Mini Waffle Maker. At that point, I spooned out portion of the chaffle player onto the waffle iron. This chaffle taco formula makes two chaffles. You can without much of a stretch twofold or triple the formula to make more at once.

Keto Chaffle in the scramble smaller than usual waffle creator cooked

When you pour the hitter on the waffle creator, close the top and don't contact for 4 minutes. I attempted to check mine part of the way through cooking and nearly discarded it as it looked as though it wasn't going to set up appropriately. It needs the full four minutes to get a decent brilliant dark colored shading and to fresh appropriately.

When the Taco Chaffle shells were done, I turned over a biscuit container and collapsed them fifty-fifty between two tins. As they cooled, they remained looking like a taco shell.

Are these Chaffle Taco Shells Crispy?

Truly! They are overly firm. They aren't eggy at all either. This Taco Chaffle formula makes incredibly crunchy taco shells that aren't oily by any stretch of the imagination.

For the flavorful ground hamburger taco meat, I recommend utilizing my most established girl's formula for the Very Best Taco Meat with my custom made keto-accommodating taco flavoring. This formula is the best taco meat I've at any point eaten. It has so a lot of mind blowing striking flavor. I in every case twofold the formula so we can appreciate it for lunch for a few days or freeze for some other time. On the off chance that you lean toward chicken, this slow cooker formula for Low Carb Mexican Shredded Chicken would be phenomenal also.

Blessed smokes, the Taco Chaffle Recipe was delectable!! It made an ideal low carb firm taco shell that we've all been absent.

Garnishes for Taco Chaffles

There are such huge numbers of keto low carb well-disposed choices for fixing Keto Taco Chaffles. I've incorporated those I could consider beneath:

harsh cream

guacamole

lettuce

destroyed cheddar

diced onions

diced tomatoes

jalapeños

Taco Chaffle formula with ground hamburger, lettuce, and cheddar

Would i be able to Make This Easy Keto Recipe Ahead of Time?

You could unquestionably make the Keto Chaffle Taco Shells early just as the taco meat. In any case, I would recommend not rewarming the taco shells in the microwave as they would lose their freshness. Rather, I envelop by aluminum foil and rewarm in the broiler or pop them noticeable all around fryer.

More Keto Chaffle Recipes:

Exceptionally Popular Traditional Keto Chaffle Recipe

Chocolate Chip Chaffle Keto Recipe

Pizza Chaffle Keto Recipe

Keto Pumpkin Keto Waffle Recipe (Chaffle)

Blueberry Keto Chaffle

Keto Chaffle Breakfast Sandwich with almond flour

Scaled down Keto Pizza with Chaffle Pizza Crust (almond flour)

Strawberry Shortcake Chaffle Recipe

Keto Chaffle Taco Shells Recipe with almond flour

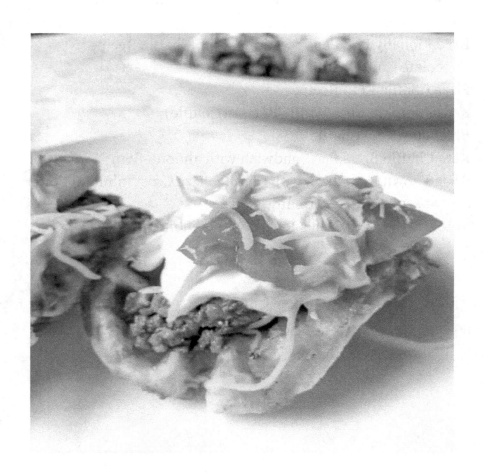

LOADED CHAFFLES NACHOS

Fixings

2 eggs

1 cup mozzarella

1/2 cheddar (I included this, you can include another cheddar)

2 TBSP Almond flour

1 tsp garlic

1 jalepeno diced

2 strips bacon

Garnishes (pick one or all)

Taco meat

Harsh cream

Guacamole

Olives

Salsa

Jalapeno cuts

Onions

Steps

Blended fixings, at that point cook in waffle producer. At the point when concocted tear or use kitchen scissors to cut up.

Layer dish with chaffles, mozzarella, cheddar, more jalapenos and taco meat. I included sweet banana peppers too.

Cook in 425 degree stove for 10 minutes or more on the off chance that you need a crisper base.

Notes

Nourishment Facts (garnishes excluded, change your macros dependent on fixings you include)

Servings: 4

Sum per 1 serving

Calories   202
Absolute Fat 15.6g
Absolute Carbohydrate 2.7g
Dietary Fiber 0.8g
Absolute Sugars 0.5g
Protein 13.4g

MOZZARELLA PANINI

Fixings

4 crusty bread sandwich rolls

2 tablespoons olive oil

1/2 cup basil pesto

8 cuts mozzarella cheddar

1 medium tomato, cut into 8 slim cuts

1/2 teaspoon salt

1/4 teaspoon pepper

Steps

1 Warmth shut contact flame broil 5 minutes.

2 Cut each move down the middle on a level plane; brush outside of every half with oil. Spread pesto on within the two parts. Layer each sandwich with cheddar and tomato. Sprinkle with salt and pepper.

3 At the point when barbecue is warmed, place sandwiches on flame broil. Close flame broil; barbecue 4 minutes or until bread is toasty and cheddar is dissolved. Cut sandwiches on corner to corner and serve warm.

Master Tips

On the off chance that you can't discover crusty bread moves, you can substitute focaccia or 8 cuts of nation bread.

This sandwich is particularly scrumptious when made with huge beefsteak tomatoes at their pinnacle of readiness. At the point when ready tomatoes are not accessible, take a stab at utilizing cleaved cherry tomatoes. They are all the more dependably delightful regardless of what the season.

New mozzarella can be utilized rather than the cuts.

PIZZA CHAFFLE

Fixings

FOR PIZZA CHAFFLES:

2 huge eggs

2 tbsp. almond flour

1/2 tsp. legitimate salt

1/2 tsp. preparing pop

1/2 c. destroyed mozzarella, separated

1/3 c. pepperoni cuts

Newly ground Parmesan, for serving

Bearings

Preheat waffle creator as per maker's headings. In a medium bowl, whisk eggs, almond flour, salt, and preparing soft drink together. Include 1 cup mozzarella and mix to cover.

Pour 1/2 cup blend into focal point of waffle creator and cook until brilliant and fresh, 2 to 3 minutes. Rehash with residual hitter.

Promptly top with marinara, remaining ½ cup mozzarella, pepperoni, and a sprinkle of Parmesan.

KETO AVOCADO AND SALMON SALAD

This serving of mixed greens makes certain to leave you full until dinnertime. The base of this plate of mixed greens is a happy spring blend close to smoked salmon, which is one of my number one augmentations to any keto serving of mixed greens as it contains a high measure of fats and great protein. The salmon is actually the way in to this formula. It is then finished off with avocado cuts and onion to give the plate of mixed greens a firm crunch.

The plate of mixed greens dressing incorporates a scramble of sugar with mustard and white wine vinegar. It is an ideal pair between sweet yet impactful, which slices through this serving of mixed greens pleasantly.

Yields 2 servings of Keto Avocado Salmon Salad

THE PREPARATION

Plate of mixed greens:

4 ounce spring blend

6 ounce smoked salmon

1 medium avocado, cut

1/2 medium red onion, cut

Plate of mixed greens Dressing:

2 tablespoon white wine vinegar

2 tablespoon olive oil

1 teaspoon dijon mustard

1 teaspoon fueled erythritol

1/2 teaspoon lemon juice

Salt and pepper to taste

Prosciutto Manchego Grilled Salad

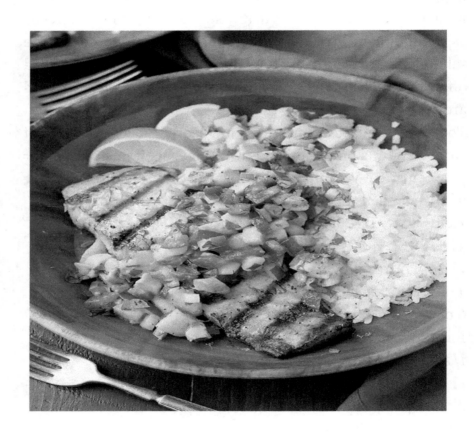

PROSCIUTTO MANCHEGO GRILLED SALAD

Warm plates of mixed greens are consistently an incredible method to flavor up standard servings of mixed greens. The lettuce in this formula is barbecued to an ideal burn on the flame broil. It is then slashed up into reduced down pieces and finished off with an Italian top pick, prosciutto.

As these ingredients are different from your normal serving of mixed greens, I realized a light dressing was expected to try to this dish is integrated magnificently. Olive oil, lemon juice, and mayonnaise were my straightforward ingredients for the dressing, which slices totally through the new, warm, barbecued lettuce.

Yields 2 servings of Keto Prosciutto and Manchego Grilled Salad

THE PREPARATION

16 ounce romaine lettuce

1/4 cup olive oil, isolated

3 ounce prosciutto

3 ounce manchego cheddar

1/2 medium lemon, juice

2 tablespoon mayonnaise

Salt and pepper to taste

THE EXECUTION

1. Measure out and set up all the ingredients. Preheat the flame broil for around 20 minutes on low warmth.

2. Cut the lettuce head down the middle. Brush the two sides of the lettuce with a large portion of the olive oil.

3. Spot lettuce on the flame broil and barbecue for a couple of moments on each side while leaving the barbecue top open. Barbecue until the external leaves are scorched.

4. Shave the manchego cheddar with a vegetable peeler or sharp knife. Hack the lettuce and prosciutto up into reduced down pieces.

5. In a bowl, consolidate the lettuce pieces with the remainder of the olive oil, mayonnaise, and lemon juice. Throw to consolidate.

6. Finish the plate of mixed greens off with the prosciutto and manchego. Season with salt and pepper.

This makes an aggregate of 2 servings of Keto Prosciutto and Manchego Grilled Salad. Each serving comes out to be 642 calories, 56.8g fat, 4.8g net carbs, and 24.1g protein.

HOT SHRIMP AVOCADO SALAD

This plate of mixed greens makes certain to cause your tastebuds to feel the warmth! It is stuffed with protein and great fats, is filling, and delectably zesty! The hot part is the shrimp, which is cooked with bean stew glue and garlic. A ginger dressing completes the serving of mixed greens magnificently. The ginger, soy sauce, and lime juice in the dressing slice through the zesty shrimp and appetizing vegetables for a classy keto-accommodating serving of mixed greens.

Yields 4 servings of Spicy Shrimp Avocado Salad

THE PREPARATION

Shrimp Salad:

2 medium avocado

1/2 medium lime, juice

5 ounce cucumber

2 ounce child spinach

2 ounce cherry tomato, cut

3 tablespoon olive oil, for broiling

1 teaspoon new garlic, minced

1 tablespoon stew glue

10 ounce shrimp, stripped

Ginger Dressing:

1/4 cup olive oil

1 tablespoon new ginger, minced

1/2 medium lime, juice

1/2 tablespoon soy sauce (or coconut aminos)

1 teaspoon new garlic, minced

Salt and pepper to taste

Keto Salad Sandwiches

These plate of mixed greens sandwiches are a pleasant method to have an invigorating and great sandwich without all the cards. The fresh tasting romaine lettuce is the base for these "sandwiches." These are then finished off with new avocado and cucumber cuts alongside cherry tomatoes. The best piece of these sandwiches is the high-fat "dressing," spread and cream cheddar. These taste so great on the lettuce leaves and give it that ideal measure of something else!

I can hardly wait to make these for lunch!

Yields 2 servings of Keto Salad Sandwiches

THE PREPARATION

2 ounce romaine lettuce

2 ounce cream cheddar

2 tablespoon spread

1/2 medium avocado

4 ounce cherry tomatoes, cut

1/4 medium cucumber, cut

1 ounce parmesan cheddar, shaved

THE EXECUTION

1. Measure out and set up all the ingredients.

2. Wash and dry the lettuce. Spread it out on a plate, this will be the base of your sandwich.

3. In a bowl, consolidate the cream cheddar and margarine. Combine completely.

4. Spread the cream cheddar and margarine blend onto the lettuce leaves.

5. Top with avocado cuts, cherry tomatoes, cucumber cuts, and parmesan cheddar.

6. Serve and appreciate!

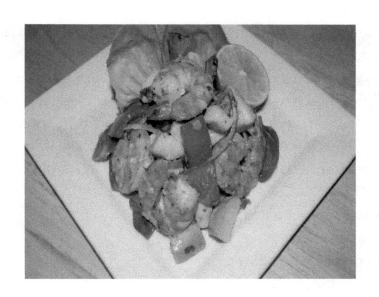

FIRM BRUSSEL SPROUT SALAD WITH LEMON DRESSING

I appreciate a decent plate of mixed greens, yet at times I don't want to have lettuce, spinach, or a spring blend as the base. I like the smash of lettuce and the flavor of spinach, however I needed to have a go at something new. Brussels sprouts end up being the ideal base for this serving of mixed greens. Indeed, you can eat Brussels sprouts crude and they taste generally excellent thusly!

On top of this serving of mixed greens is a tasty walnut and seed mixture. The walnuts, pumpkin and sunflower seeds are singed in a fiery and tart stew glue close by cumin with a scramble of salt. The lemon dressing marinates the Brussels fledglings to soften them up, and afterward is finished off with the walnut and seed blend to give a crunchy and tasty lunch or side!

Yields 4 servings of Keto Crispy Brussel Sprout Salad

THE PREPARATION

For Brussel Sprout Salad:

1 tablespoon olive oil

1 teaspoon bean stew glue

2 ounce walnuts

1 ounce pumpkin seeds

1 ounce sunflower seeds

1/2 teaspoon cumin

Salt to taste

16 ounce brussel sprouts

For Lemon Dressing:

1/2 cup olive oil

1 medium lemon, squeeze and zing

Salt and pepper to taste

THE EXECUTION

1. Accumulate and prep all ingredients.

2. In a skillet on low to medium warmth, heat up the olive oil and the bean stew glue.

3. Add the walnuts to the hot skillet and mix well.

4. Mix in the pumpkin and sunflower seeds. Season with cumin and salt. Saute for a couple of moments, blending every so often, until the walnuts and seeds are softly cooked and smells fragrant.

5. Flush the Brussels fledglings and shave them by cutting them into slight cuts with a sharp knife. Spot them in a bowl.

6. Make the lemon dressing by joining olive oil, lemon squeeze and zing, and salt and pepper to taste. Pour this over the brussel sprouts in the bowl and let this marinate for 10 minutes.

7. Before serving, include the walnut and seed blend and throw to join.

8. Finish off with extra salt and pepper if wanted. Appreciate! This makes an aggregate of 4 servings of Keto Crispy Brussel Sprout Salad. Each serving comes out to be 485 calories, 46.2g fat, 10.1g net carbs, and 7.2g protein.

HALLOUMI SALAD WITH MINT DRESSING

This halloumi cheddar plate of mixed greens with mint dressing is extraordinary for veggie lovers, cheddar darlings, and anybody needing a touch of something Greek.

If you don't have a clue what halloumi cheddar is yet, it is a staple in Greek cooking. It's a firm cheddar that doesn't liquefy making it ideal for flame broiling and serving warm. Browning the halloumi cheddar in this formula sets it consummately with new, fresh blended greens and the mint dressing served on top. The mint dressing sets so well with the halloumi, adding some tang and newness to slice through the rich greasy cheddar. The Greek yogurt, new mint, new garlic, and olive oil draw out the halloumi considerably more, making for an excessively invigorating plate of mixed greens.

Need more halloumi plans? Look at this halloumi sandwich.

Yields 4 servings of Keto Halloumi Salad with Mint Dressing

THE PREPARATION

10 ounce halloumi cheddar

1 cup full fat plain greek yogurt

1/4 cup new mint, cleaved

2 tablespoon olive oil

1 teaspoon garlic, cleaved

Salt and pepper to taste

10 ounces blended greens

1 medium lemon

THE EXECUTION

1. Accumulate and prep all ingredients.

2. In a bowl, join greek yogurt, new mint, new garlic, olive oil, and salt and pepper. Mix until consolidated well and put in a safe spot.

3. Put the halloumi cheddar into a nonstick skillet without oil or margarine. Fry on medium warmth for 2-4 minutes. Apply strain to the center of the cheddar prior to turning to guarantee the center of the cheddar is getting cooked.

4. Flip the halloumi cheddar over and do likewise to this side until the cheddar is brilliant earthy colored in shading. Eliminate from the skillet cautiously.

5. Put blended greens into a serving bowl and add the halloumi cheddar on top. Press the lemon on top and present with the mint dressing.

This makes a sum of 4 servings of Keto Halloumi Salad with Mint Dressing. Each serving comes out to be 354 calories, 25.8g fat, 7.1g net carbs, and 22.7g protein.

BARBECUED TUNA SALAD WITH GARLIC DRESSING

This serving of mixed greens is as acceptable if worse than the manner in which it looks! New barbecued fish on a bed of greens with onion, cherry tomatoes, and hard-bubbled eggs. For added surface and flavor, we sprinkle cleaved pecans and shower with a garlic dressing. This is one stuffed serving of mixed greens!

The new flame broiled fish is an incredible option in contrast to canned fish, bringing a tasty flavor that you can't get from a can. With a decent measure of fat and protein in this keto serving of mixed greens, it will assist you with remaining more full for quite a long time to come. This is an incredible feast for lunch or supper!

Yields 2 servings of Keto Grilled Tuna Salad

THE PREPARATION

2 huge egg

8 ounce asparagus lances

1 tablespoon olive oil

8 ounce new fish

4 ounce spring blend

2 ounce cherry tomatoes

1/2 medium red onion

2 tablespoon pecans, hacked

1/2 cup mayonnaise

2 tablespoon water

2 teaspoon garlic powder

Salt and pepper to taste

THE EXECUTION

1. Accumulate and prep all ingredients.

2. In a bowl, set up mayonnaise, water, garlic powder, and salt and pepper to make the dressing. Mix until joined well and put in a safe spot.

3. Heat up the eggs for around 8-10 minutes. When cooled, strip and cut down the middle.

4. Wash and cut the asparagus into equivalent lengths. Fry the asparagus in a skillet without help from anyone else.

5. Similarly pour the olive oil on the two sides of the new fish and fry for 3-5 minutes on the two sides. Season the fish with salt and pepper, to taste.

6. On a plate, place the verdant greens, cherry tomatoes (cut down the middle), onion, and eggs.

7. Cut the flame broiled fish into cuts and spot on top. Pour the dressing on top of the serving of mixed greens and sprinkle the hacked pecans in addition.

This makes an aggregate of 2 servings of Grilled Tuna Salad. Each serving comes out to be 743 calories, 58.4g fat, 9.8g net carbs, and 40.9g protein.

RICH KETO TACO SOUP

Keto taco soup might be the ideal soup formula. It's anything but difficult to-make, especially fulfilling, and can be adjusted to the Crock-Pot or Instant Pot without any problem. (Additionally, you can make it cooler amicable for an overly brisk keto supper.)

Notwithstanding, there's one trick — We'll need to skirt the beans, corn, and tortilla chips that are often hiding in taco soup. With this keto taco soup formula, they won't be fundamental in any case.

Is Taco Soup Good for Keto?

However long you skirt the beans, corn, and tortilla chips, you're well headed to a keto-accommodating soup. The taco preparing may likewise accompany covered up carbs, so ensure it's good for keto also (like this formula).

To take the fat substance and flavor past what you'd get from a standard taco soup, we additionally suggest utilizing some hefty cream and high-fat ground hamburger rather than lower-fat ingredients.

Basically, these are altogether the progressions you'll need to make for the ideal keto taco soup, regardless of whether you cook it in the moderate cooker, on your burner, or in your moment pot.

Three Ways to Make Keto Taco Soup: Stovetop, Crock-Pot, or Instant Pot

With the formula ventures beneath, we stayed with the most available cooking strategy: the burner. Notwithstanding, it is anything but difficult to make this in your moderate cooker or Instant Pot too:

Keto Taco Soup in the Crock-Pot Slow Cooker

Essentially earthy colored the hamburger on the burner, then add it to the moderate cooker with the entirety of different ingredients. Cook on high for 3-4 hours or on low for 6 hours.

Moment Pot Keto-accommodating Taco Soup

Utilizing the saute capacity on your Instant Pot, earthy colored the hamburger and cook the onions and garlic. Then, add and blend in the excess ingredients.

Physically set the tension on high for 10 minutes with common delivery.

How Long Does Keto Taco Soup Last? Capacity Options for the Fridge and Freezer

Your keto taco soup will keep going for as long as 4 days in a hermetically sealed holder in the cooler. (Following a day or two in the cooler, I discover the soup tastes surprisingly better!)

You can likewise freeze the taco soup (prior to adding any embellishments). Just freeze each serving in an impenetrable compartment for as long as a half year. For ideal newness, eat it inside a quarter of a year.

What Can I Serve With My Keto Taco Soup?

Other than adding the toppings from the ingredients list beneath, here are some other keto-accommodating alternatives you can attempt with your soup:

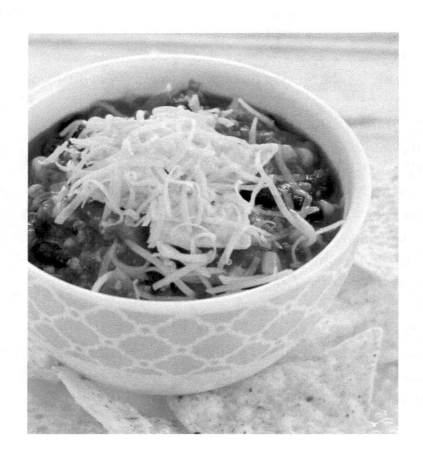

KETO TORTILLA CHIPS

Garlic and Herb Breadstick Bites

A cut of Keto Bread with spread

A low-carb side plate of mixed greens

Keto Grilled Cheese

Garlic Parmesan Keto Croutons (to add some bread-like surface to the soup)

Would i be able to Make Keto Taco Soup With Chicken Instead of Beef?

Indeed, you can. Don't hesitate to utilize any meat you'd like.

Ground chicken or turkey will work best, yet you can likewise utilize pulled rotisserie chicken or chicken thigh meat.

If you're hoping to change things up much more with different flavors and surfaces, check these keto chicken soup plans out also:

Moment Pot King Ranch Chicken Soup

Slow cooker Buffalo Chicken Soup

Chicken Enchilada Soup

Yields 6 servings of Keto Taco Soup

THE PREPARATION

For Soup:

16 ounce ground hamburger

1 tablespoon olive oil

1 medium onion, diced

3 cloves garlic, minced

1 medium green ringer pepper, diced

10 ounce canned tomatoes with green chile

1 cup weighty cream

2 tablespoons taco preparing (formula here)

Salt and pepper to taste

2 cups meat stock

To Garnish:

1 medium avocado, cubed

4 tablespoons sharp cream

4 tablespoons cilantro, hacked

THE EXECUTION

1. Accumulate and prep all ingredients. Dice the onion and ringer pepper early.

2. In a pot over medium warmth, add olive oil, onion, garlic, and ground meat. Season with salt and pepper.

3. Cook until meat is carmelized and onion is clear.

4. When the meat is carmelized, include the ringer pepper, diced tomato with green chile, weighty cream, and taco preparing.

5. Mix together well trying to join the flavoring through the entirety of the ingredients.

6. Include the meat stock and afterward heat soup to the point of boiling. When bubbling, diminish to low and stew for 10-15 minutes, or until fluid has decreased and soup is thickened to your inclination. Taste and season with salt and pepper if wanted.

7. Bit out servings and topping with avocado, harsh cream, and cilantro. A crush of lime juice is incredible, as well!

This makes an aggregate of 6 servings of Keto Taco Soup. Each serving comes out to be 470 calories, 37.1g fat, 6.7g net carbs, and 24.7g protein.

KETO CHICKEN SALAD

Chicken plate of mixed greens is extraordinary compared to other keto staples. With the correct ingredients, it checks all the cases for an ideal keto-accommodating dinner: fulfilling, tasty, solid, advantageous, and flexible.

The solitary issue is that all chicken plates of mixed greens aren't made the equivalent. Some are too rich, some have an excess of vinegar, and others accompany superfluous high-carb ingredients.

Finding the correct equilibrium of flavors and surfaces is a test, so we chose to take chicken serving of mixed greens to the keto kitchen for a makeover. The outcome left me puzzled (generally because I was unable to shield myself from taking another nibble).

Is Chicken Salad Keto?

It relies upon what sort of chicken serving of mixed greens you are having. Exemplary chicken plate of mixed greens — with mayo, celery, red onion, chicken, and a little dijon mustard — is keto-accommodating.

In any case, when you toss in any new or dried organic product, for example, craisins, apples, or grapes, there will be an excessive number of carbs in your chicken serving of mixed greens for keto. This is the reason is ideal to stay with a keto-endorsed formula for chicken serving of mixed greens that you realize will hit the detect without fail.

Top Tips for Making the Best Keto Chicken Salad

In the wake of trying different things with many different chicken plate of mixed greens plans throughout the long term, I've discovered that these three hints to give the most blast to the buck:

Add avocado. The avocado gives it some additional smoothness without making it excessively rich. It additionally furnishes us with an incredible method to sneak in some extra solid fats, fiber, minerals, and nutrients.

Utilize chicken thigh, not bosom. Chicken thighs have more fat and flavor, making them the ideal meat for keto chicken serving of mixed greens. Also, they are a lot less expensive than chicken bosoms.

Remember the hard-bubbled eggs. The novel surfaces from the hard-bubbled yolk and whites gives the chicken plate of mixed greens another measurement that keeps it fulfilling through the last nibble.

Step by step instructions to Store Your Keto Chicken Salad

If you're seeking dinner prep for the week or store any extras, put every chicken plate of mixed greens serving in an impermeable holder in the ice chest.

By putting away it thusly, you can have snappy and flavorful keto suppers that will remain new for as long as seven days.

What Else Can I Add To My Keto Chicken Salad

Chicken serving of mixed greens is flexible to the point that you can make it a different way each time and never get exhausted of it.

If you're hoping to add another degree of flavor or surface to your chicken serving of mixed greens, attempt these keto-accommodating options:

Wild ox sauce and disintegrated blue cheddar (to make a Buffalo chicken serving of mixed greens)

Slashed Fire and Ice Pickles

Destroyed cheddar

Keto-endorsed farm (supplant a portion of the mayo with farm)

Slashed fresh bacon

1/8 – 1/4 tsp of bean stew powder

Slashed walnuts (or other low carb nuts)

Or on the other hand take a stab at exchanging up the vast majority of the formula with our Keto Venezuelan Chicken Salad.

What to Serve with Your Keto Chicken Salad

Despite the fact that it is too fulfilling by the forkful, here are some alternate approaches to overhaul your keto chicken serving of mixed greens dinner:

Make a chicken plate of mixed greens sandwich with keto cloud bread

Attempt a chicken serving of mixed greens dissolve with cheddar and 90-second keto bread

Wrap it up with romaine or spread lettuce

Transform it into a chicken plate of mixed greens wrap with keto tortillas

Serve on top of your #1 low carb plate of mixed greens

Spread it on keto wafers or cucumber cuts

Plunge keto tortilla chips or cheddar chips into it

What's your #1 method to have a chicken plate of mixed greens? Tell us in the remarks underneath.

Yields 4 servings of Keto Chicken Salad

THE PREPARATION

8 ounce chicken thighs, cooked and cubed

2 enormous eggs, hard-bubbled to your inclination

2/3 cup mayonnaise

1 medium avocado

1 tablespoon lime juice

1/4 medium red onion, diced

1 stem celery, diced

salt and pepper, to taste

1/4 cup cilantro, to decorate

4 low carb tortillas, locally acquired or natively constructed [recipe here]

THE EXECUTION

1. Assemble and prep all ingredients. Hard-heat up the eggs and cook the chicken if required.

2. In a food processor or blender, consolidate the mayonnaise, lime juice, and half of the avocado. Season with salt and pepper to taste.

3. 3D shape the leftover portion of the avocado and slash the hard-bubbled eggs.

4. In a bowl, consolidate the chicken, onion, celery, avocado, egg, and mayonnaise dressing. Season with extra salt and pepper to taste.

5. Combine until consolidated and dressing is covering all ingredients equitably. Spot in the cooler until prepared to serve.

6. Toast tortilla up in a container, then serve the cool chicken plate of mixed greens over the top. Trimming with cilantro, if wanted.

This makes a sum of 4 servings of Keto Chicken Salad. Each serving comes out to be 539 calories, 46.4g fat, 6.5g net carbs, and 21.1g protein.

MUSHROOMS AND GOAT CHEESE SALAD

Wow – this is one stunning plate of mixed greens! The best part is the mushrooms sauteed in margarine. It helps keep the lettuce wet and matches well with the balsamic vinegar dressing and disintegrated goat cheddar.

Mushrooms and Goat Cheese Salad

For this formula I utilized a child greens blend from the store however if you can't find that combination even infant kale, spinach, and a little romaine will go far with this scrumptious dish. On the other hand for the cheddar, you could likewise attempt pieces of brie or feta. Each would taste similarly as delicious.

Need to make it for work? Simply keep the balsamic vinegar discrete and it should be acceptable in the cooler for as long as 3 days.

Yields 1 serving of Mushrooms and Goat Cheese Salad

THE PREPARATION

1 tablespoon margarine

2 ounces cremini mushrooms, cut

Salt and pepper, to taste

4 ounces spring blend

1 ounce cooked bacon, disintegrated

1 ounce goat cheddar, disintegrated

1 tablespoon balsamic vinegar

1 tablespoon olive oil

Natively constructed Keto Caesar Salad

Here's the way you can make an exemplary Caesar serving of mixed greens at home, with keto-accommodating ingredients. We add a lot of Parmesan cheddar and dressing however skirt the bread garnishes for firm bacon. If you've just got extra chicken available, then you could make this for lunch instantly by any means.

Natively constructed Keto Caesar Salad

The dressing utilizes anchovy filets, giving it that exemplary flavor profile, however if you can't stand them then don't hesitate to skip it. Another tip is that if you can discover jolted anchovies then utilize those rather than canned because then you won't need to stress over spending the extra filets immediately. You can just reseal the container.

Yields 2 servings of Homemade Keto Caesar Salad

THE PREPARATION

Serving of mixed greens

10 ounces boneless, skinless chicken bosom

1 tablespoon olive oil

Salt and pepper, to taste

2 ounces cooked bacon

8 ounces romaine lettuce

1 ounce Parmesan cheddar, ground

Dressing

½ cup mayonnaise

1 tablespoon Dijon mustard

½ medium lemon, zing and juice

½ ounce Parmesan cheddar, ground

2 tablespoons finely slashed anchovy filets

1 teaspoon minced garlic

Salt and pepper, to taste

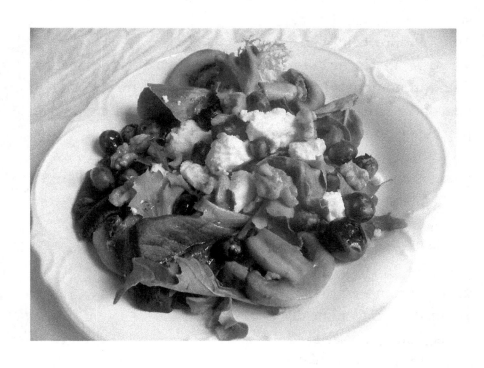

TART KETO BROCCOLI SALAD

What could be superior to this tart broccoli serving of mixed greens with bacon, cheddar, pumpkin seeds, and a tart dressing? It's an incredible plate of mixed greens or side dish, however since it requires no cooking, it's additionally simple to get ready. The vast majority could never see that this is low carb, so it's an extraordinary formula to bring when you need something to share!

Tart Keto Broccoli Salad

There's some erythritol in the dressing to supplant the sugar found in numerous broccoli serving of mixed greens plans. If you don't care for a better dressing, then don't hesitate to preclude it altogether. If you're not ready to eat dairy, then you could likewise avoid the cheddar, and it would even now be extraordinary. As should be obvious, this plate of mixed greens is adaptable and can be effortlessly changed to suit your preferences.

Yields 8 servings of Tangy Keto Broccoli Salad

THE PREPARATION

2.5 pounds broccoli, cut into reduced down pieces

1/2 medium red onion, diced

1/2 cup pumpkin seeds

4 ounces cheddar, cubed

3/4 cup mayonnaise

5 tablespoons erythritol

3 tablespoons apple juice vinegar

Salt and pepper, to taste

6 ounces cooked bacon, disintegrated

THE EXECUTION

1. In a bowl, join the broccoli, diced red onion, pumpkin seeds, and cubed cheddar.

2. In a different bowl, join the mayonnaise, erythritol, and apple juice vinegar.

3. Add the mayonnaise combination into the plate of mixed greens and mix well. Season with salt and pepper to taste then place into the cooler for at any rate 3 hours.

4. Add the disintegrated, cooked bacon prior to serving.

This makes a sum of 8 servings of Tangy Keto Broccoli Salad. Each serving comes out to be 386.75 Calories, 30.73g Fats, 8.33g Net Carbs, and 15.24g Protein.

KETO WARM KALE SALAD

Kale leaves seared in margarine then threw with Dijon mustard dressing, and finished off with disintegrated feta cheddar. The dressing is my new most loved approach to eat kale, and there's something truly fulfilling about getting into a bowl that is both sound and heavenly. This generous plate of mixed greens works extraordinary as a supplement pressed side dish for supper, or basically as lunch.

Keto Warm Kale Salad

This is another extraordinary base formula that you can cause your all own occasions you to make it. Different garnishes you should attempt incorporate bacon, keto bread garnishes, cleaved ham, barbecued chicken, or even hard-bubbled eggs.

Yields 2 servings of Keto Warm Kale Salad

THE PREPARATION

Warm Salad

2 tablespoons margarine

4 ounces kale

2 ounces feta cheddar

Salt and pepper, to taste

Dressing

4 tablespoons weighty whipping cream

1 teaspoon mayonnaise

1 teaspoon dijon mustard

½ teaspoon garlic

THE EXECUTION

1. Mix the weighty cream, mayonnaise, Dijon mustard, and garlic together until smooth. Put in a safe spot.

---

2. Flush the kale and hack into reduced down pieces. Dispose of the stem.

3. Add the margarine to a dish over medium warmth. When hot, add the kale to the container and rapidly cook until a dim earthy colored shading comes out. Around 1-2 minutes.

4. Spot cooked kale into a bowl. Top with feta cheddar and dressing. Season with salt and pepper to taste.

This makes a sum of 2 servings of Keto Warm Kale Salad. Each serving comes out to be 343 Calories, 33.7g Fats, 4.3g Net Carbs, and 6.25g Protein.

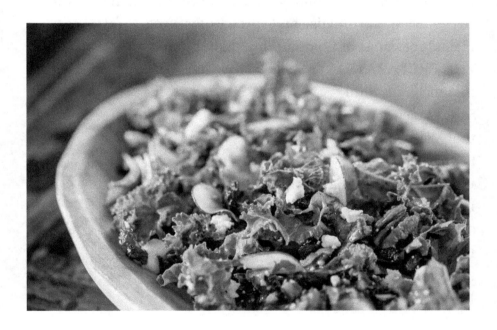

COLD ZUCCHINI SALAD

This cool zucchini plate of mixed greens is the ideal summery serving of mixed greens for serving close by BBQ. We make this with sauteed zucchini, celery, loads of onion, and a mayonnaise-based dressing. This serving of mixed greens is extraordinary for making ahead because it's surprisingly better if you let it sit for the time being.

There's no compelling reason to break out the spiralizer or even the vegetable peeler because the zucchini is essentially slashed, which gives it an incredible thick surface. Have a go at adding some rotisserie chicken and feta cheddar for a heartier turn. It's veggie lover of course and can be made vegetarian if you utilize a vegetarian mayonnaise and spread substitute.

Yields 3 servings of Cold Zucchini Salad

THE PREPARATION

16 ounces zucchini

Salt, to taste

1 tablespoon margarine

Pepper, to taste

1.5 ounces celery, cut

1 ounce green onion, slashed

0.5 cups mayonnaise

1 tablespoon slashed chives

1 teaspoon Dijon mustard

THE EXECUTION

1. Strip the zucchini and afterward cut fifty-fifty length-wise. Utilize a spoon to scratch out the seeds of the zucchini. Cleave zucchini into half-inch cuts. Spot the zucchini in a colander with salt to draw the water out. Leave for 5-10 minutes and afterward softly press remaining water out of the zucchini.

2. Rapidly sautee the zucchini in a container with spread over medium warmth. Season with salt and pepper to taste. Cook the zucchini until marginally softened, around 2-3 minutes. Eliminate from the warmth and put aside to cool.

3. When the zucchini is cooled, combine the excess ingredients into a bowl and serve.

This makes an aggregate of 3 servings of Cold Zucchini Salad. Each serving comes out to be 469 Calories, 47.8g Fats, 5.2g Net Carbs, and 3.7g Protein.

The Preparation

16 ounces zucchini

Salt, to taste

1 tablespoon spread

Pepper, to taste

1.5 ounces celery, cut

1 ounce green onion, cleaved

0.5 cups mayonnaise

1 tablespoon cleaved chives

1 teaspoon Dijon mustard

The Execution

1. Strip the zucchini and afterward cut into equal parts length-wise. Utilize a spoon to scratch out the seeds of the zucchini. Slash zucchini into half-inch cuts. Spot the zucchini in a colander with salt to draw the water out. Leave for 5-10 minutes and afterward delicately press remaining water out of the zucchini.

2. Rapidly sautee the zucchini in a skillet with spread over medium warmth. Season with salt and pepper to taste. Cook the zucchini until somewhat softened, around 2-3 minutes. Eliminate from the warmth and put aside to cool.

3. When the zucchini is cooled, combine the excess ingredients into a bowl and serve.

Notes

This makes a sum of 3 servings of Cold Zucchini Salad. Each serving comes out to be 469 Calories, 47.8g Fats, 5.2g Net Carbs, and 3.7g Protein.

KETO ASPARAGUS, EGG, AND BACON SALAD

An asparagus serving of mixed greens finished off with bacon and eggs, then dressed with a tart dijon vinaigrette. The dressing is effectively made with storeroom staples that you probably have close by. That makes it incredible for preparing any time you discover extraordinary asparagus.

You can save time by making extra hard-bubbled eggs or bacon when you cook them for different plans. That way, you should simply whiten the asparagus and make the dressing. I like to have both in my refrigerator consistently.

Yields 2 servings of Keto Asparagus, Egg, and Bacon Salad

THE PREPARATION

Serving of mixed greens

16 ounces asparagus lances

3 ounces bacon

2 enormous hard-bubbled eggs, cleaved

Dressing

2 tablespoons avocado oil

2 tablespoons red wine vinegar

1 tablespoon dijon mustard

1 teaspoon minced garlic

½ teaspoon squashed red pepper pieces

Salt and pepper, to taste

THE EXECUTION

1. Trim the asparagus, then cleave into 1-2 inch portions.

2. Carry a pot of salted water to bubble. Add the asparagus into the pot and bubble for 3-4 minutes. Utilize an opened spoon to eliminate the asparagus from the bubbling water and move to a bowl loaded up with ice water to stop the cooking cycle.

3. Hack the bacon into little pieces and afterward cook in a skillet over medium warmth until delivered and fresh.

4. Add the entirety of the dressing ingredients into a bowl alongside the bacon fat from the container that you cooked the bacon in. Whisk together vivaciously to consolidate. Season with salt and pepper.

5. Amass the serving of mixed greens by consolidating the asparagus, bacon, slashed hard-bubbled eggs, and dressing. Combine and serve.

This makes a sum of 2 servings of Keto Asparagus, Egg, and Bacon Salad. Each serving comes out to be 481 Calories, 39.4g Fats, 5.35g Net Carbs, and 23.05g Protein.

KETO HOAGIE LUNCH BOWL

This simple lunch bowl joins all your number one flavors from a Hoagie roll, however with no of the bread. We slash up virus cuts like turkey, salami, and ham then throw it with a lot of cheddar and veggies and sauce.

You can hack the ingredients and blend the sauce previously for quick and simple snacks. Next to no prepare and no cooking is required. I think, similar to me, you'll additionally conclude that you don't miss the bread. It's difficult to miss it when you can at present eat the very best pieces of the sandwich!

Yields 4 servings of Keto Hoagie Lunch Bowl

THE PREPARATION

Bowl

4 ounces cooked turkey, hacked

4 ounces Italian dry salami, slashed

4 ounces store cut dark backwoods ham, hacked

4 ounces Provolone cheddar, cubed

2 ounces sharp cheddar, cubed

2 ounces destroyed spring blend lettuce

2.5 ounces cherry tomatoes, slashed

3.5 ounces cucumber, cubed

1 ounce banana peppers, hacked

0.25 medium red onion, diced

Sauce

4 tablespoons mayonnaise

2 tablespoons red wine vinegar

1 tablespoon olive oil

0.5 teaspoon dried basil

0.75 teaspoon Italian flavoring

Salt and pepper, to taste

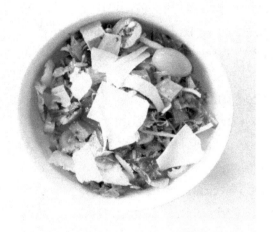

CPSIA information can be obtained
at www.ICGtesting.com
Printed in the USA
LVHW021026220121
677169LV00012B/358